Chest and Shoulders

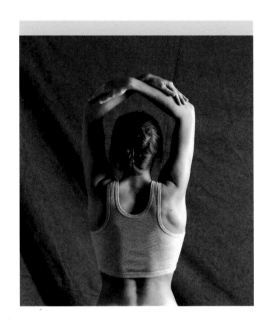

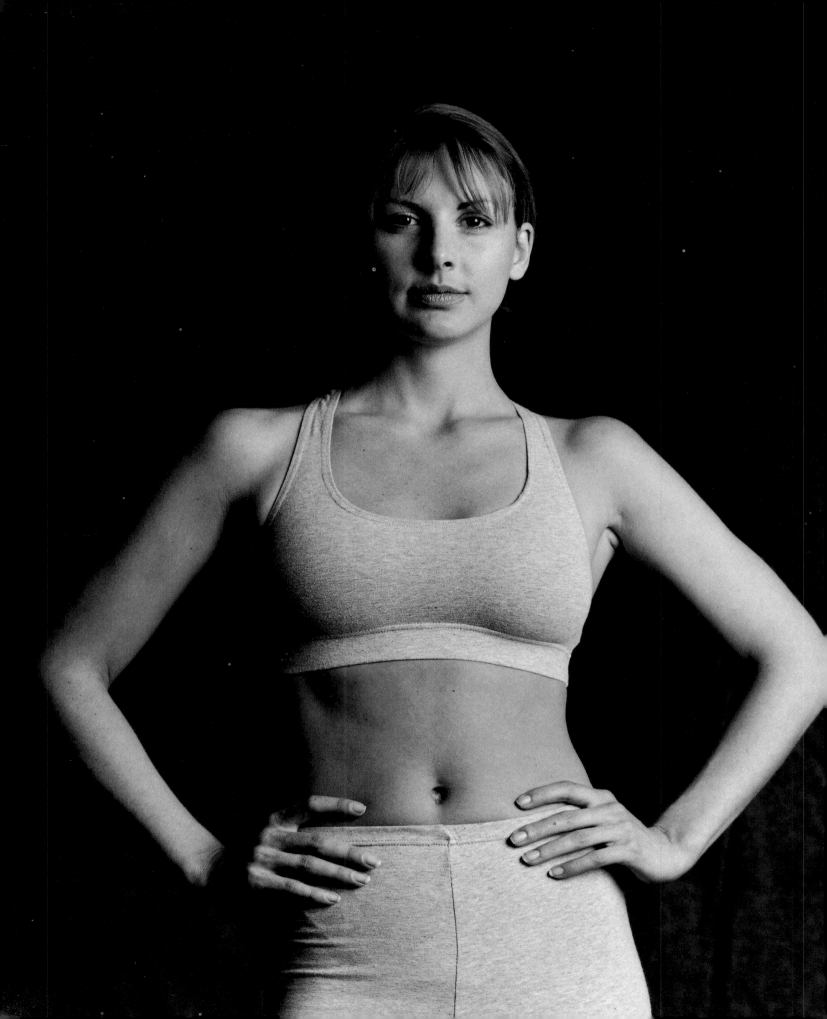

The Supple Workout

Chest and Shoulders

Catherine McCrum

Photography by Antonia Deutsch

MACMILLAN • USA

MACMILLAN
A Simon and Schuster Macmillan Company
1633 Broadway
New York, NY 10019

A DBP Book
conceived, created and designed by
Duncan Baird Publishers
Sixth Floor
Castle House
75–76 Wells Street
London W1P 3RE

A catalogue record is available from the Library
of Congress.
ISBN 0-02-861345-7

Designers: Sue Bush, Gail Jones
Editor: Stephanie Driver
Commissioned Photography: Antonia Deutsch

10 9 8 7 6 5 4 3 2 1

Typeset in Frutiger
Colour reproduction by Bright Arts, Hong Kong
Printed in Singapore

Publishers' note
The exercises in this book are intended for
healthy people who want to be fitter. However,
exercise in inappropriate circumstances can be
harmful, and even fit, healthy people can injure
themselves. The publishers, DBP, the author, and
the photographer cannot accept any
responsibility for any injuries or damage
incurred as a result of using this book.

Contents

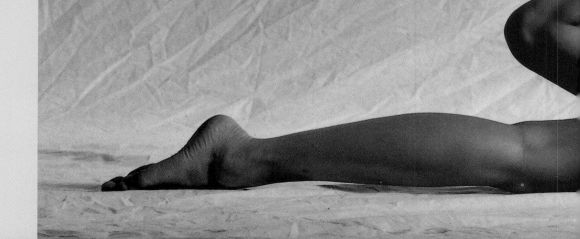

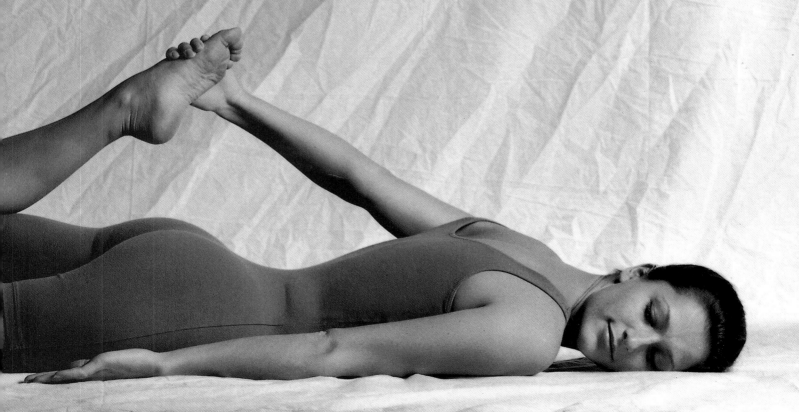

Introduction

A strong and upright torso with a broad chest suggests confidence. Tension in the chest pulls the shoulders forward, creating a hunched posture, which is not only unattractive, but also unhealthy, since it restricts lung capacity.

It is easy to make a simple program of regular exercise an integral part of a healthy lifestyle. You will soon start to benefit from a renewed sense of energy and vitality and from a more toned and attractive body.

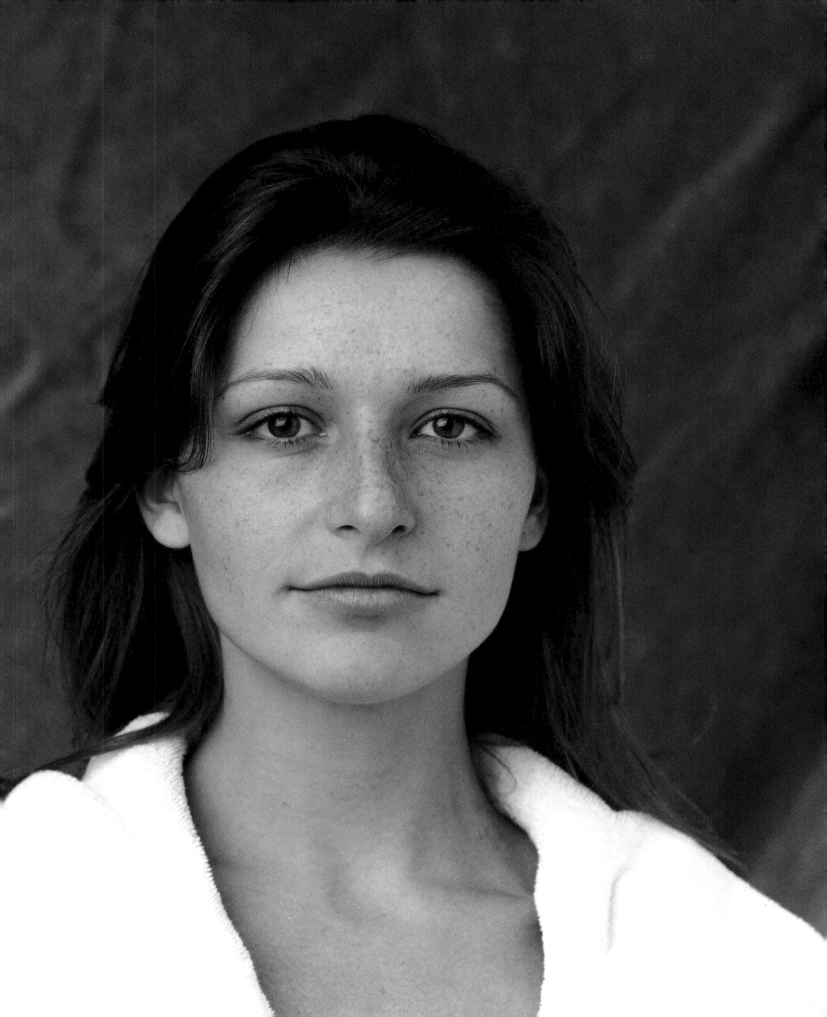

Getting started:
how to use this book

A complete chest and shoulder workout includes strength and stretch exercises for both the front and back of the upper body. For balance, it also includes exercises for the waist and abdomen.

After a few weeks of regular exercise, you will begin to notice improvement in your muscle tone – your back should feel looser, your neck and shoulders more relaxed. After four to six weeks your abdomen should be firmer and your chest and shoulders will be more open. Your improved posture will make you appear taller and more confident.

Do not attempt an advanced variation of an exercise until you are confident that you can perform the basic exercise correctly. Use weights to increase the difficulty as suggested only when you can comfortably complete all the repetitions of the basic stage. Wear training shoes if you are using weights.

The exercises should be performed slowly and with control. You should feel mild tension in the muscles that you are stretching – sharp pain is your body's warning mechanism.

Always try to breathe smoothly and calmly throughout each repetition of an exercise. It is usual to breathe out on the exertion phase of an exercise and breathe in during the relaxation phase.

The recommended repetitions are just guidelines. Work at your own pace, building up the number of repetitions slowly and gently, rather than risk injury by doing too much. Listen to your body and do what feels right for you. Some days that may be less, other days you may have more energy.

Before you begin, do a posture check. Stand side on to a mirror with your abdominals drawn in and your shoulders and chest open and upper back broad. Try to lengthen your body from your heels to the top of your neck. Ideally, your ears, shoulders, hips, knees, and ankles should be in a direct line. Turn to the front. Your knees and feet should be lined up parallel with each other and facing forward, your weight should be balanced evenly across both legs and feet, and your hips and shoulders should be parallel to the floor.

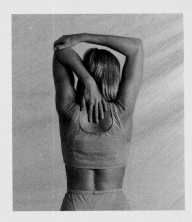

Core exercises, pages 22–45
These exercises will teach you how to develop a balanced torso, with strong and flexible muscles in your chest, shoulders, and abdomen. Strength moves are complemented by stretches, so you will develop a long, lean line, not bulk.

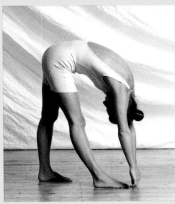

Warm-ups and cool-downs, pages 46–55
Before you begin exercising, it is essential to spend a few minutes warming up, to avoid the chance of injury. It is just as important to spend a few minutes cooling down at the end, returning your body to its normal, relaxed state.

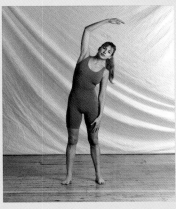

Total body workout, pages 56–67
These exercises targeting the back, hips, and thighs will complement the core exercises, allowing you to tone your whole body in a balanced, healthy manner. Exercises for the back are the essential counterpoint for front-of-the-body work, and those for the hips and thighs enhance the condition of your lower body.

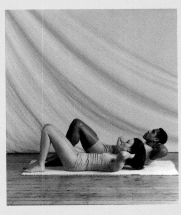

Routines, pages 68–77
How you combine exercises to create a routine will depend on your mood, your energy level, and how much time you want to spend. These two sample routines are great examples of the different types of combinations you can put together on your own.

Complete fitness:
the components of health

Whether it was concern for your health or concern for your appearance that first got you interested in exercising your chest and shoulders, it is important to understand the role any exercise plays in a plan for total health and fitness.

By toning your chest and shoulder muscles, you will achieve greater balance in your upper body. Your chest muscles work in opposition to the muscles of your upper back, so if they are tight, your posture inevitably suffers. Your shoulders become rounded and your chest concave, pulling your back out of alignment. This restricts the size of your lung cavity, as your rib cage is not able to expand to its full capacity. Once you begin the exercises in this book, you will soon notice your improved posture and freer breathing, and you will feel stronger and more energetic.

But improving the condition of your chest and shoulders is only one aspect of an overall fitness plan. That is why this book presents a Total Body Workout, so you can tone your entire body at the same time as you focus on your chest and shoulders. The aim of any sensible exercise plan is to achieve balance in your physical state.

Exercise is obviously one of the keys to health and fitness, but it is only one part of the equation for a fit and toned body. A healthy diet is an equally important contributor to your overall well-being – and to a more vibrant appearance.

As soon as you understand the simple, basic principles of healthy eating, you will see that it is easy to make it an integral part of your day-to-day life.

The table opposite is the template you need to plan your meals and snacks. A healthy diet is not a question of counting calories – balance is the key. Each day, you should plan your meals and your snacks around a selection of good foods taken from the full range of food groups. You will get all the nutrients you need, and you will soon look and feel better.

A little advance planning is especially useful when it comes to snacking. In a recent poll, 75 per cent of people admitted to snacking between meals. When you are trying to watch what you eat, the midday (or midnight) snack is dangerous territory. By planning ahead, you will be able to make sure that you have plenty of low-fat, nutritious possibilities on hand.

Daily nutrition

Food groups	What counts as a serving?	Recommended per day
1 Grain products group (bread, cereal, rice, and pasta)	• 1 slice of bread • 1 ounce (30 grams) of ready-to-eat cereal • 1/2 cup of cooked cereal, rice, or pasta	6–11 servings
2 Vegetable group	• 1 cup of raw leafy vegetables • 1/2 cup of other vegetables • 3/4 cup of vegetable juice	3–5 servings
3 Fruit group	• 1 medium apple, banana, orange • 1/2 cup of cooked or canned fruit • 3/4 cup of fruit juice	2–4 servings
4 Milk group (milk, yogurt, and cheese)	• 1 cup of milk or yogurt • 1 1/2 ounces (40 grams) of natural cheese • 2 ounces of processed cheese	2–3 servings
5 Meat and beans group (meat, poultry, fish, dry beans, eggs, and nuts)	• 2–3 ounces (60–90 grams) of cooked lean meat, poultry, or fish • 1/2 cup of cooked dry beans or 1 egg counts as 1 ounce of lean meat • Two tablespoons of peanut butter or 1/3 cup of nuts count as 1 ounce of lean meat	2–3 servings

Source: USDA

Some foods fit into more than one group. "Crossover" foods, such as dry beans, peas, and lentils, can be counted as servings in either the meat and beans group or vegetable group, but not both in the same meal. This makes things easy for vegetarians.

Don't be intimidated by the number of servings in the grains category – the portions are smaller than most people generally have, so you if have double the amount of pasta for dinner, that counts as two of your grain servings.

Once you understand these principles, it is simple to lose weight if you want to. The table gives a range of recommended servings, and you should follow the lower number in the range, choosing lower-fat alternatives and preparing your food using little oil and butter.

Because it is not a restrictive diet, you can easily fit it into your day-to-day life, continuing to eat out in restaurants or at friends' homes.

Remember that muscle weighs more than fat. When you combine diet with exercise, you will

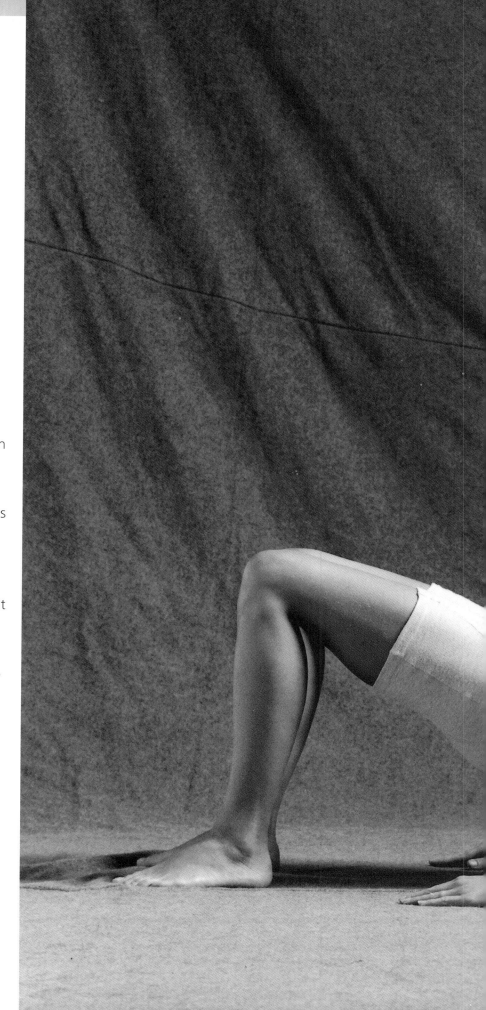

be losing fat at the same time as you are building up muscle. The results may be more impressive in the mirror than on the scales.

The elements of physical fitness

Just as you need to learn the basic principles of healthy eating to plan your diet, it is important to understand the different components of physical fitness in order to plan your exercise.

Flexibility – the ability of the joints and muscles to achieve their full range of motion – is one. The exercises in this book will enhance the flexibility of your chest and shoulder muscles: after only a few sessions, you will notice that it is easier to complete the exercises correctly.

By toning these muscles, you will also improve their endurance – the ability of the muscles to sustain repeated force or action. It is easy to notice improvements in endurance – with practice, you will be able to complete more repetitions of an exercise.

Strength – the ability of muscles to exert force for short periods of time – is another component of fitness, which is why there are many strength exercises in this book. Most

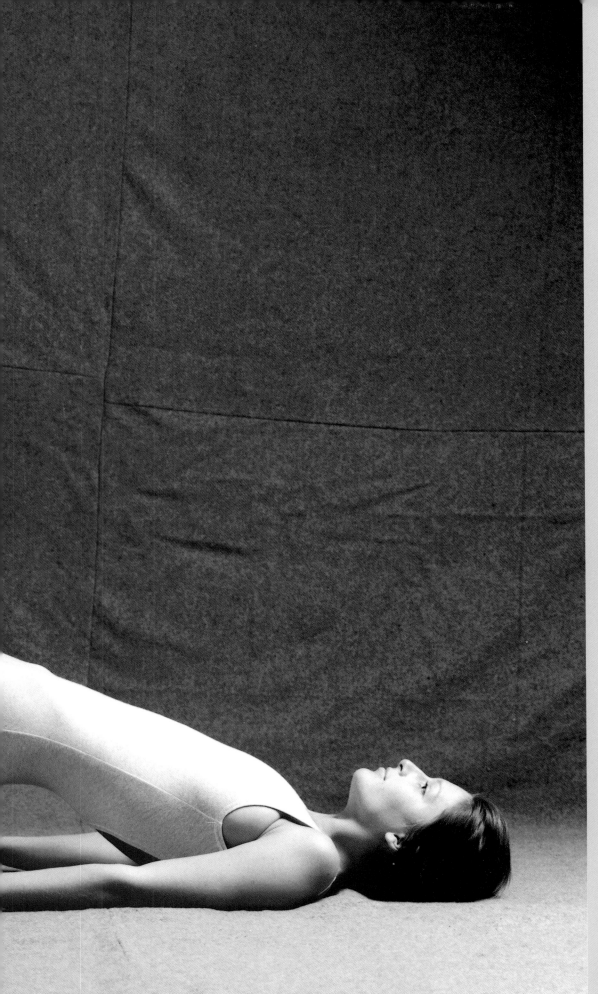

For a healthy, toned body, you must balance diet with exercise. Experts recommend that you do around 30 minutes of moderate exercise at least five days a week – you can break the 30 minutes up into smaller blocks of time throughout your day if that is easier for you. Cardiovascular exercise, such as fast walking, cycling, or jogging, is an important component of any exercise plan. It increases your metabolic rate not just when you are working out, but also for some time afterward, so you will continue to burn calories. Note that for cardiovascular exercise to be effective, you must sustain a raised heartrate continuously for 20 minutes or more.

involve muscles working against the force of gravity, but the most effective way to increase strength is to work with weights. A number of the exercises in this book can be enhanced with the use of weights. While flexibility exercises will help you to tone your muscles, strength exercises will help you to increase their size. As you progress to heavier weights, you will start to notice a gradual change. When working with weights, always wear training shoes.

Cardiovascular fitness is also an essential attribute of a healthy body. This refers to the ability of the body to produce enhanced blood flow that will supply additional oxygen and nutrients to active tissues and remove the metabolic waste products.

Any form of aerobic exercise that improves the ability of the heart to pump more blood will contribute to cardiovascular fitness: this includes forms of exercise such as brisk walking, running, cycling, or swimming, all of which cause a sustained, raised heartrate. Aerobic exercises will also help to improve your muscle tone.

Exercise is like dieting – you are not likely to continue with an exercise program that is time-consuming and complicated. However, there are a few basic principles for exercise, just as there are for diet.

Exercise experts recommend 30 minutes of moderate exercise at least five days a week. This sounds like a lot, until you take into consideration the fact that you do not have to do it all at once. Three ten-minute blocks of gentle strength and stretching exercises are just as effective as a dedicated half-hour (cardiovascular exercise is an exception – it is essential to sustain a raised heartrate for 20 to 30 minutes).

The best advice for overall fitness is also the simplest. Try to make your lifestyle more active: take the stairs instead of the elevator, and walk to the shops instead of driving once in a while. The changes are simple, but the benefits are vast.

Women tend to have less upper body strength than men do. By doing the exercises in this book, they can benefit from toning and strengthening their chest and shoulders, without worrying about developing bulging muscles. On the other hand, men, by adding weights, can work to develop their musculature.

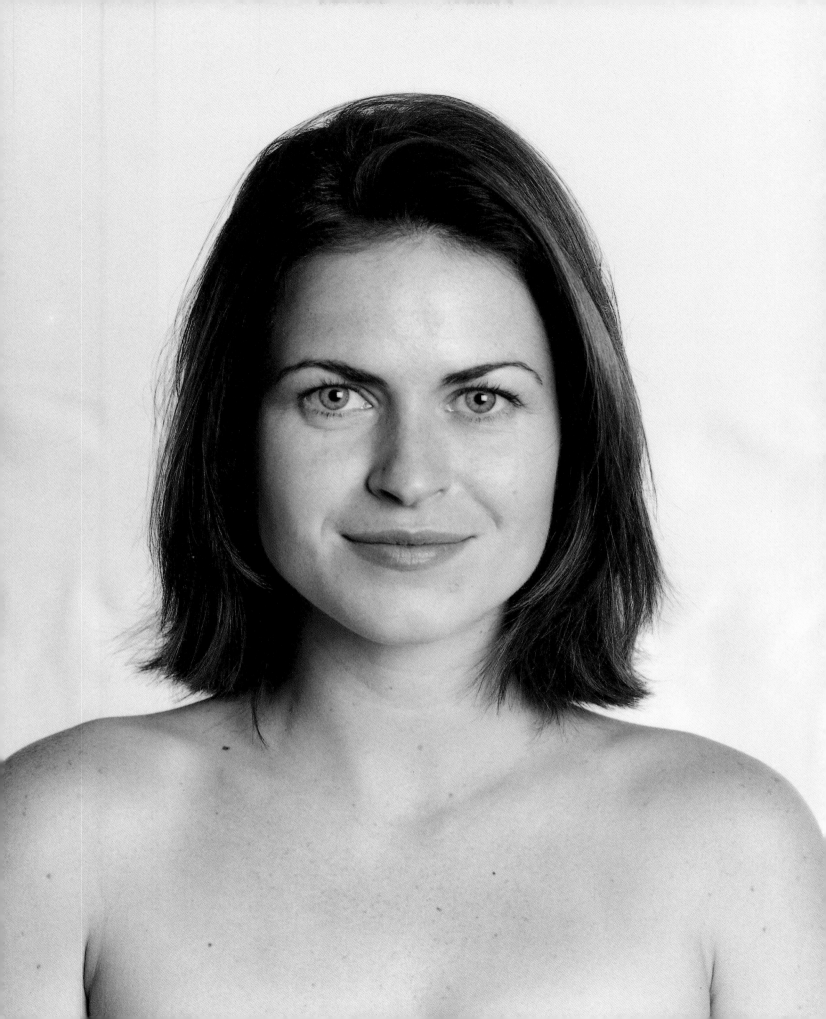

Body facts

The muscles of the chest and shoulders are essential in many everyday activities, including lifting and carrying, typing, eating, and even breathing. Along with the abdominals and the back muscles, they work to support the torso, maintaining its stability.

In order to tone these muscles effectively by stretching and strengthening them, it is important to understand where they are, how they are inter-related, and how they work.

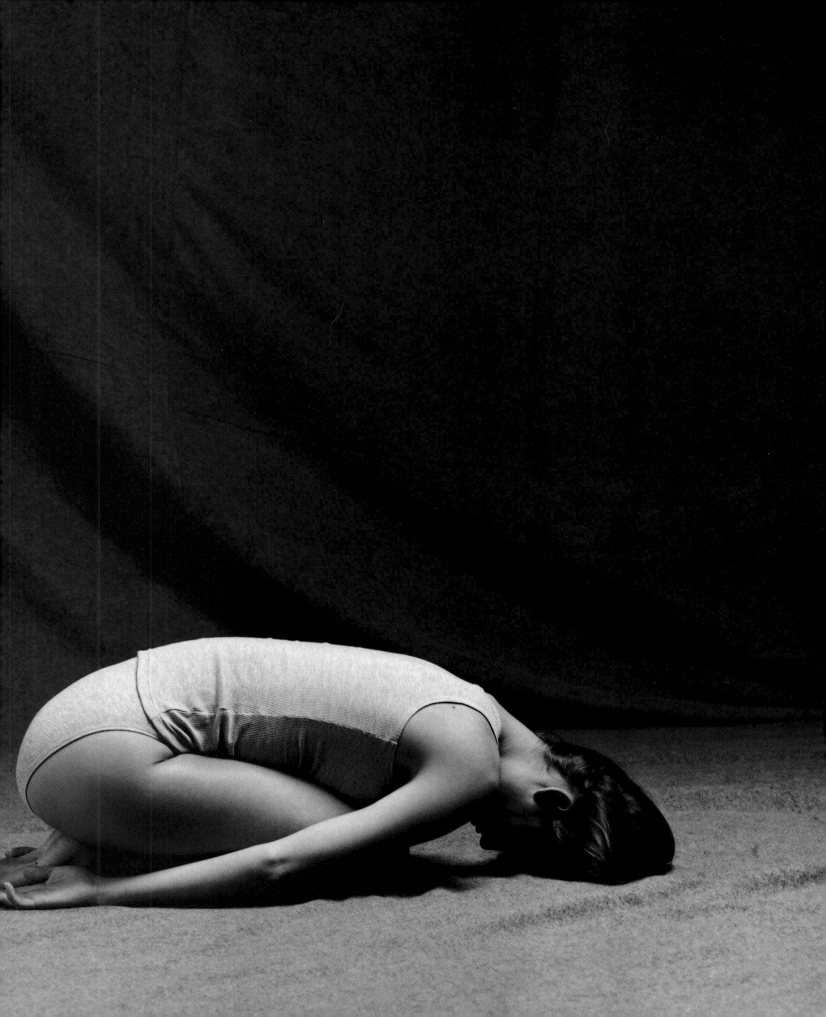

Body facts: chest and shoulders

The muscles of the chest and shoulders, and the abdominals, support the upper body, working in partnership with the muscles of the back. They are involved in many day-to-day activities, from bending to lifting, and even breathing.

The chest and shoulder muscles are anchored around the pectoral girdle, which consists of the shoulder blades (scapulae) and the collar bone (clavicle). These muscles connect the shoulder blades to the trunk; in particular, the serratus anterior keeps the shoulder blades from "winging" out. The muscles in this area work in opposition to each other: tight shoulder muscles will widen the chest abnormally; and tight chest muscles will cause the shoulders to round and hunch.

The shoulder joint is a ball-and-socket joint, which allows the arms a wide range of movement. This involves the coordination of a large number of muscles, not only in the shoulders and chest, but also in the arms and down the back. The shoulder is stabilized by the various muscles of the rotator cuff: the subcapularis, supraspinatus, infraspinatus, and teres minor. These are often weak and easily injured.

There are two muscles in the chest, commonly known as the "pecs".

The pectoralis major is the larger of the two, and it runs up the chest from the abdomen to the collar bone. It also connects to the back of the upper arm. You can exercise this muscle by doing different kinds of push-ups. It works in opposition to the deltoids in the shoulder, by moving the arms down and bringing them forward in front of the body. The deltoids run from the collar bone across the shoulder blade to the back of the upper arm. The triceps are the main muscles at the back of the upper arm, which extend the arm at the elbow, in opposition to the biceps, which bend the arm. The triceps are weak and flabby in many people.

The pectoralis minor lies under the pectoralis major, working in opposition to the trapezius muscle to bring the shoulder down and forward. The trapezius, which runs from the base of the skull, along the neck and upper spine, across the shoulder blades and to the rear of the collar bone, works to raise the arms higher than shoulder level. Along with the rhomboids, it also generally supports the shoulders and arms.

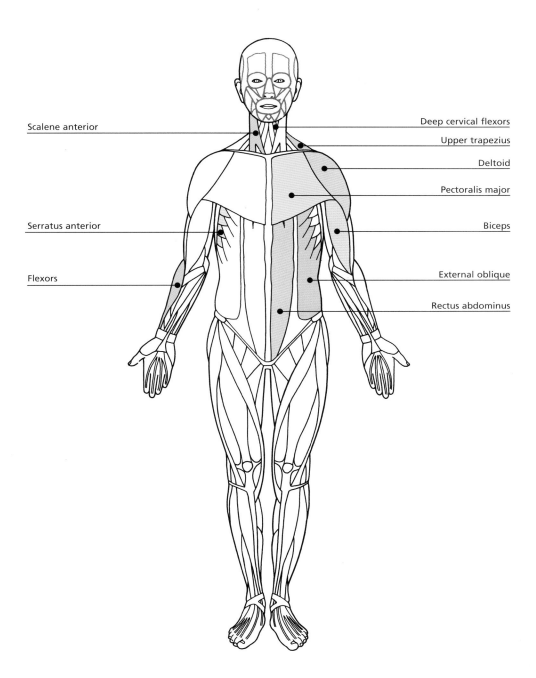

Scalene anterior

Serratus anterior

Flexors

Deep cervical flexors

Upper trapezius

Deltoid

Pectoralis major

Biceps

External oblique

Rectus abdominus

Front of the body

This diagram clearly illustrates the way in which the muscles of the front of the body are interrelated. The pectoralis major is the largest of the chest and shoulder muscles, and runs across the chest from the abdomen to the collar bone. It works in opposition to the deltoids, which run from the front of the body around to the back. Not all the abdominal muscles appear in this type of diagram, because the abs are in four layers of muscle, with the rectus abdominus on top at the front and the external obliques showing at the sides: the others are hidden.

The abdominals are a group of four different muscles. One, the rectus abdominus, runs upward on either side of the midline of the body, from the pubic bone to the ribs. The other three are flat sheets of muscle that together make up the front wall of your body. Working from the inside out, these are the transverse abdominus, the internal oblique, and the external oblique.

The grain of each runs in a different direction: the fibers of the transverse abdominus run forward and horizontally; the internal oblique runs forward and up; and the external oblique runs forward and down. On the skin surface the rectus abdominus gives the rippled appearance to well-toned abs.

Because the fibers of these muscles run in different directions, the muscles have great strength, even though they are thin. It is important to understand this when you are planning your exercise, because each muscle needs to be exercised in a specific way, working with the direction in which the fibers run. For example, to tone the rectus abdominus, you have to do curl-ups or pelvic tilts, but to tone the obliques, you need to do twisting exercises.

The abdominal muscles serve a number of purposes in the body. In terms of movement, they begin the action of bending forward from the pelvis, when you are standing or sitting; they are integral to any twisting movement; and they assist in the movement of the legs and the hips. They work against the muscles of the lower back, keeping your back from arching excessively. They form a protective wall, safely holding the internal organs, and when they contract, they help the body expel waste products. Finally, these muscles are instrumental in breathing, and therefore in speaking as well as singing.

The abdominal muscles are quick to suffer the ravages of age. They weaken and stretch, allowing the midriff to sag. In consequence, the lower back often arches, because the abdominals are not strong enough to work in opposition to the lower back muscles. This is not only unattractive – it also leads to the lower back pain that all too many people suffer from these days.

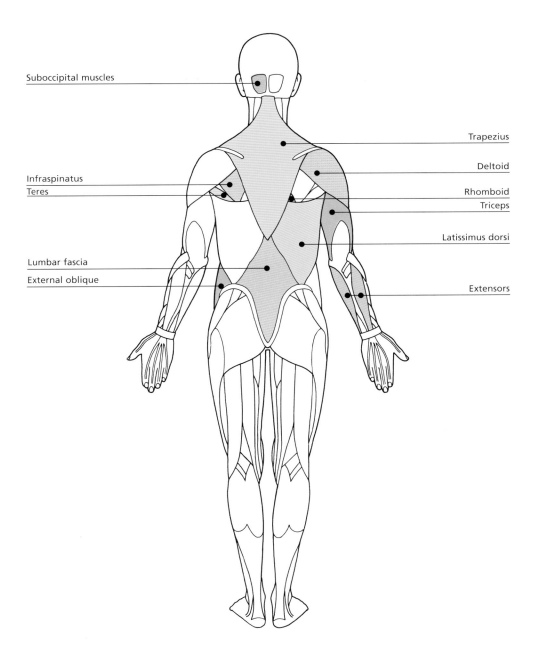

Suboccipital muscles

Infraspinatus

Teres

Lumbar fascia

External oblique

Trapezius

Deltoid

Rhomboid

Triceps

Latissimus dorsi

Extensors

Back of the body

From the rear, it is easy to see the complex arrangement of the shoulder muscles. The deltoid wraps around the shoulders from the chest to the back muscles. The external obliques, which are part of the abdominal muscle group, also wrap around to the back of the body. The muscles of the rotator cuff – the supraspinatus, infraspinatus, subcapularis, and teres minor – are essential for the stability of the shoulder joint; in many people, however, they are weak and easily injured. The shoulder muscles are also clearly related to the back and neck.

Core exercises

A balanced torso, with strong, flexible shoulders and chest, helps to safeguard against back problems and poor posture. By adding some abdominal exercises for your waist, you will develop a longer spine, a broad, open chest and shoulders, and a firmer, flatter stomach, and you will appear taller and improve your overall body shape.

There's a large number of strength-based exercises and stretches to help you develop this part of your body. In this selection, each toning exercise is placed near a stretch for the same muscle group to ensure that muscles remain long and flexible.

For the best results, you should perform a balanced selection of exercises two or three times a week. If you have less time, do two different strength exercises with their accompanying stretches daily.

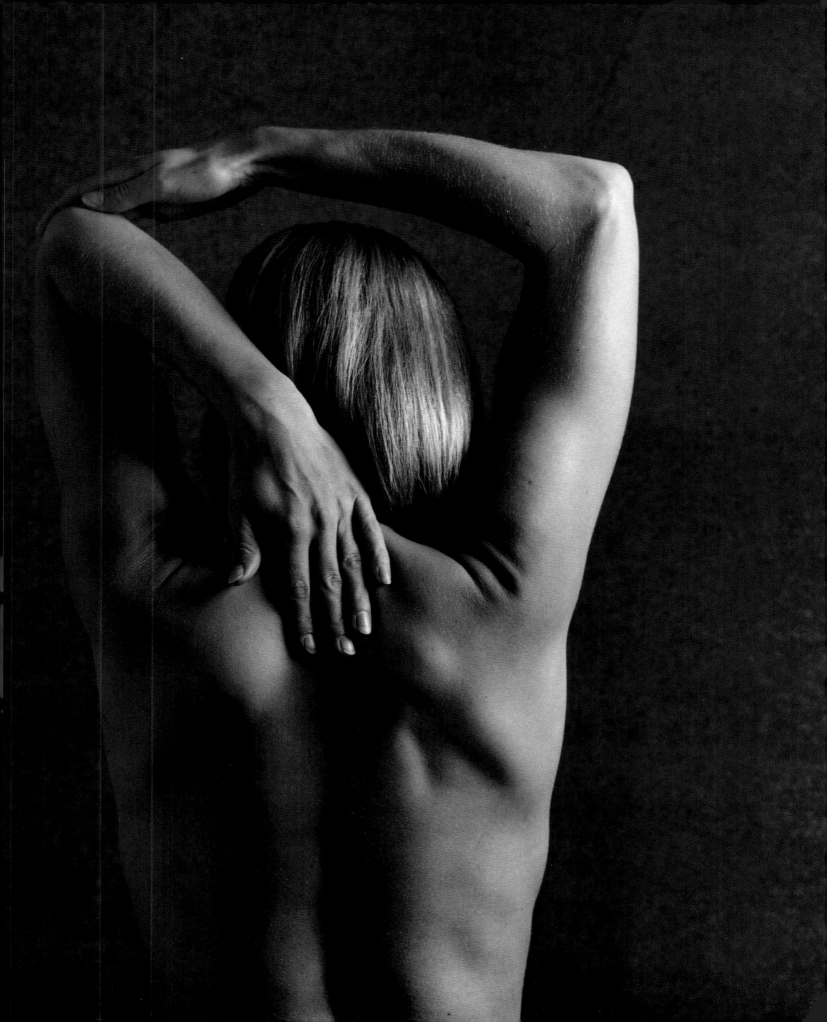

Chest and shoulders

A sedentary lifestyle can create imbalances in the chest and shoulder muscles. Tight chest muscles pull the shoulders into a rounded position, causing the upper back to stretch and weaken. This throws the head and neck forward, out of alignment with the spine. The neck and shoulder pain that results will be familiar to many people.

By stretching the tight muscles in your chest, you will open the shoulder girdle, prevent rounded shoulders, and expand the rib cage, allowing your lungs the space to breathe freely and easily. When you develop stronger shoulders, many everyday lifting and carrying activities will be easier, and your arms and upper body will have a toned appearance.

Be very aware of your posture when you do these exercises. Keep the shoulder girdle open and the shoulder blades drawn down the back. If you do an exercise for these muscles with your shoulders rounded, you will only make worse any muscular imbalances that you may already have.

❶

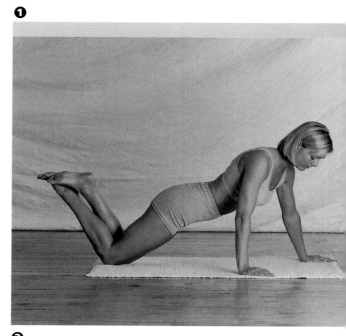

❷

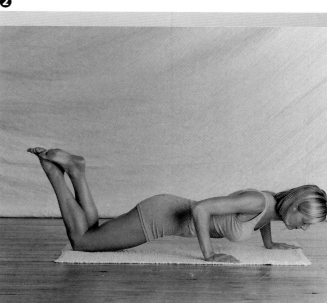

Staggered press-up
This is a variation on the classic press-up. Place your left hand on the floor in front of your shoulder and your right hand behind, slightly wider than shoulders' width apart, and establish a straight line from the top of your head through your hips to your knees, and cross your ankles (1). Keeping your buttocks tight and your navel to your spine, lower your chest to the floor by bending your elbows (2). Repeat eight to 12 times (or however many you can complete with good form) before moving the other hand to the front.

❶

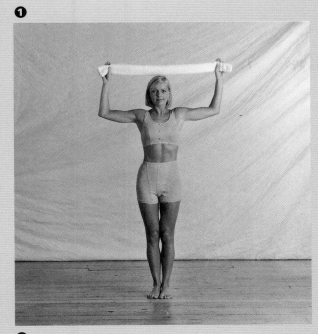

❸

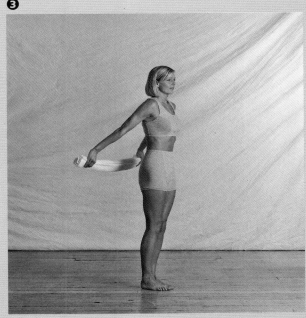

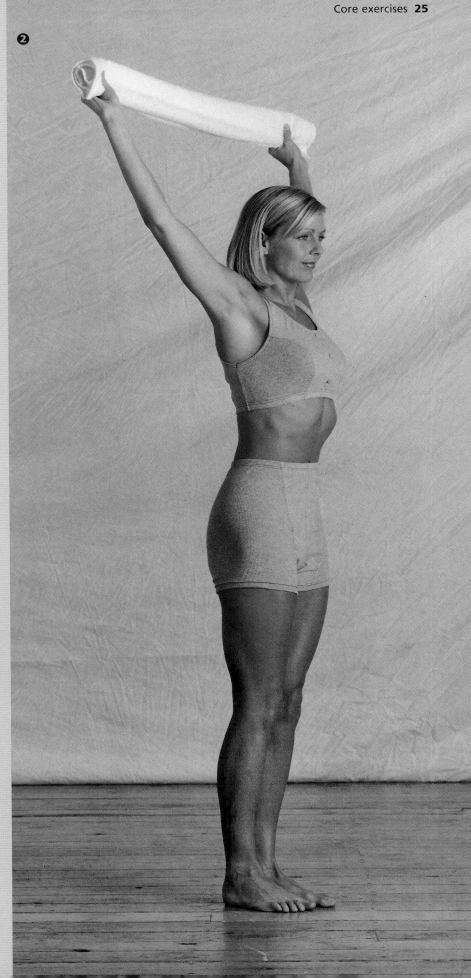

Towel stretch

This is a very deep stretch for your chest. With your arms at shoulder height, elbows bent to right angles, wrists directly above elbows, and palms facing forward, hold a towel taut between both hands (1). Extend your arms into a V shape above your head (2), then move your arms behind your body, keeping your elbows straight, until you feel a stretch in the chest and shoulders (3). Try to keep the arms moving back slowly and evenly, without poking your chin forward. Ultimately you will be able to bring your hands around and down toward your buttocks.

Ceiling pulse

This exercise works on the muscles at the back of the upper arms.

   Lying face down with your arms by your sides, palms facing the ceiling, contract your buttocks and draw your tailbone to the floor. Raise your chest off the floor, feeling the lower back contract (1). Hold this position for a few seconds. Rotate your arms to the ceiling so your palms are facing the floor, and lift your arms a small distance up and down (2), four times. Relax and lower your body to the floor, before repeating the sequence from four to eight times.

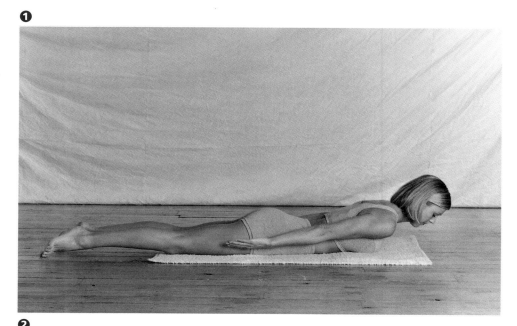

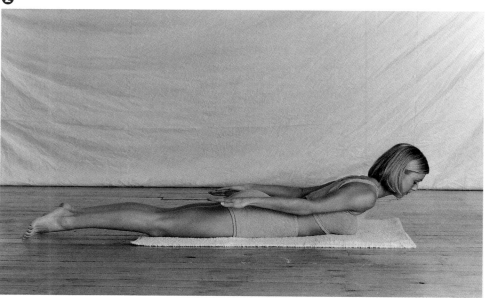

①

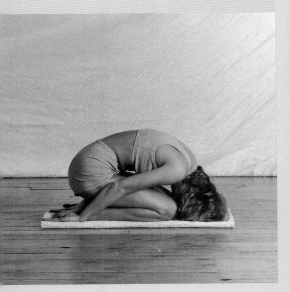

②

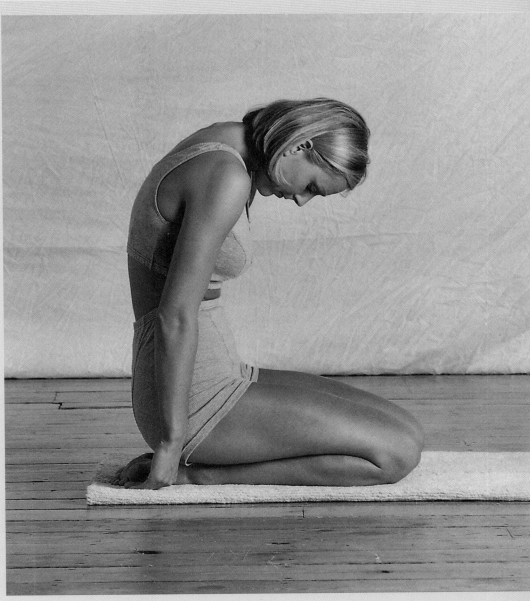

Re-stack
Kneeling with your buttocks resting on
your feet, bend over until your head rests
on the floor, allowing your arms to relax
on the floor with your hands, palms up, by
your feet (1). Relax this way for a few
moments before returning to an upright,
sitting position by rolling up through the
spine one vertebra at a time (2), leaving
your head to come up last.

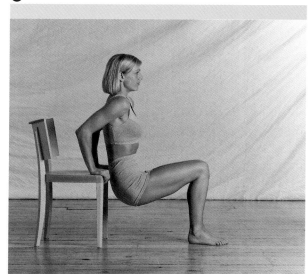

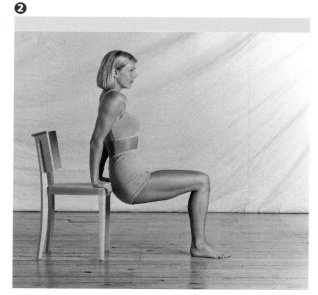

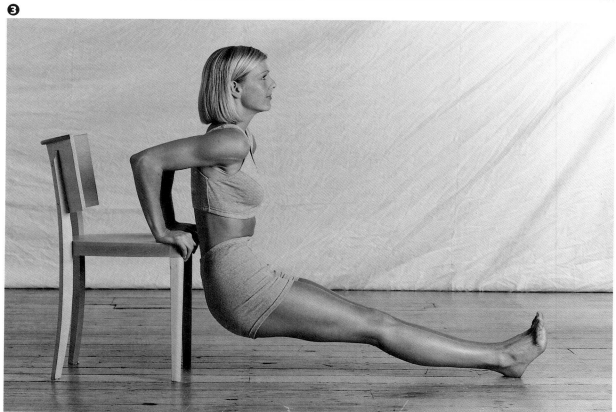

Tricep dip

Place your hands hips' width apart on a chair, your fingertips facing forward (1). Straighten your arms, keeping your back long and lowering your shoulders to draw them away from your ears, until your your knees and hips are level and your thighs are parallel to the floor (2), then bend your elbows again toward the back of the chair, lowering your body toward the floor. Make sure you draw your shoulder blades down your back to avoid strain on your neck. Repeat this sequence five times, building up to 20 repetitions. As a challenging variation, raise and lower your body with your legs straight (3).

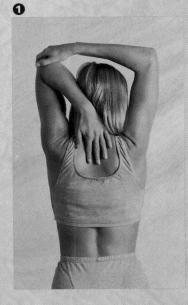

Tricep stretch

Standing, raise your left arm up to the ceiling, then bend your elbow, placing your hand between your shoulders. Clasp your left elbow with your right hand and gently try to draw the left elbow behind your head (1). Don't allow your head to drop forward as you stretch. Hold this for 20 to 30 seconds before repeating on the other side.

If you find this difficult, you can use a towel to make it gentler. Holding one end of a towel in your left hand, bend your left elbow, letting the towel drop down your back. Hold it with your right hand, inching your hand up the towel as far as you can, gently pulling your left arm down (2).

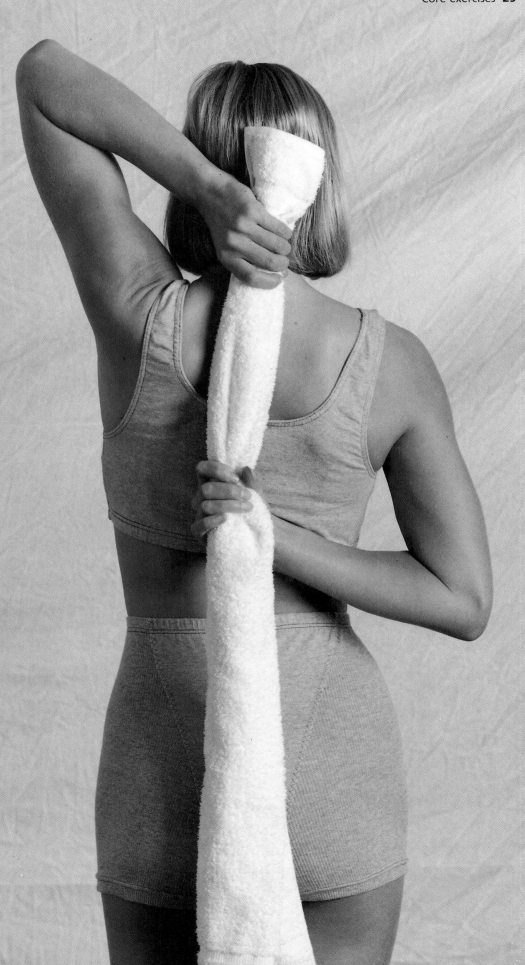

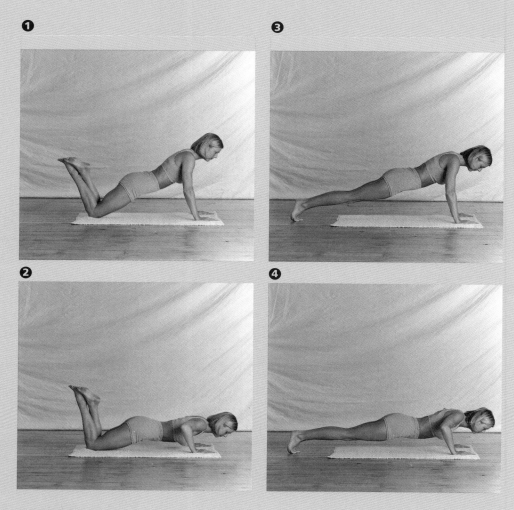

Classic press-up

This is a good over-all exercise to strengthen your chest and shoulders.

Starting on your hands and knees, with your hands wider than shoulders' width apart and your fingertips facing forward, establish a straight line from the top of your head through your hips to your knees, and cross your ankles (1). Keeping your buttocks tight and your navel to your spine, slowly lower your chest toward the floor (2). Aim to lower your chest all the way to the floor, hold for a few seconds, then raise your body. When you can do 20 with good form, try the advanced version. Keeping your body in a straight line from your heels to the top of your head (3), slowly lower your chest to the floor (4), pushing off your palms to raise your body.

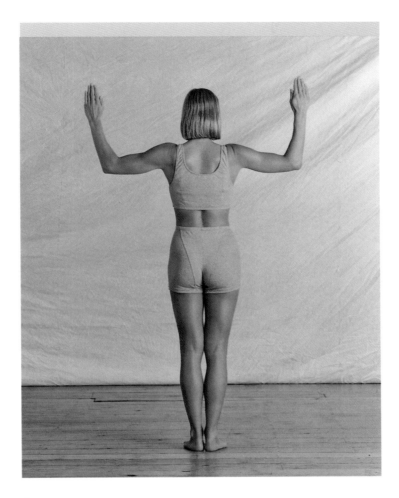

Box arms

With your arms out at shoulder height, bend your elbows to right angles with your palms facing forward. Think of anchoring your shoulder blades to your rib cage at the same time as you open your chest and shoulders. Your wrists should be directly above your elbow joint. Hold for a count of 10, rest, and repeat.

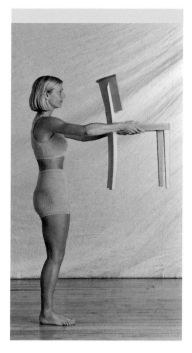 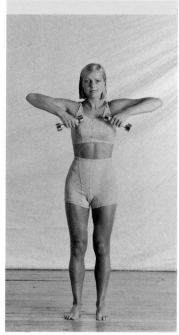 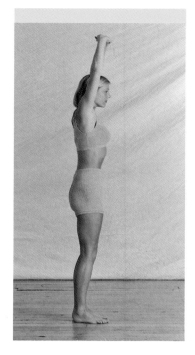

Chair lift

This strength move will work on your shoulders and your postural muscles.

Stand with your feet hips' width apart, abdominals pulled in, and your shoulder blades drawn down your back. Pick up a light chair (bending your knees as you lift), and keeping your arms shoulders' width apart with your elbows slightly bent, slowly raise the chair to shoulder height. Concentrate on keeping your spine long. Hold for five seconds before carefully lowering the chair. Repeat five times.

Upright row

Stand with your feet hips' width apart, knees soft, and stabilize your spine by drawing in your abdominals. Place your hands about six inches (15 cm) apart with your arms straight down. Slowly raise your elbows to just above shoulder height, allowing your hands to follow and making sure you don't cock your wrists. Lower your arms to the starting position. You will feel the movement in your shoulders and upper back. Repeat 12 times, building up to 20 as you grow stronger. You can use light weights if you want to increase the intensity.

Overhead reach

This is an easy and relaxing stretch. Standing with good posture, clasp your hands in front of your body with your palms facing away from you. Slowly raise your arms above your head and pull back gently until you feel a stretch in your armpits and shoulders. With practice, you should be able to draw your arms behind your ears. Be careful that your rib cage doesn't pop out and that your chin doesn't protrude.

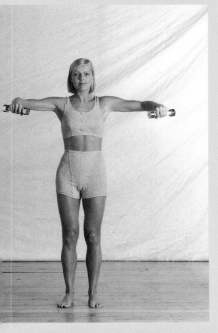

Lateral raise

Keeping your elbows slightly bent, your arms long, and palms facing the floor, smoothly raise your arms to shoulder height, performing the movement with control rather than with momentum. Make sure you do not hunch your shoulders. Lower your arms, then repeat eight times, building up to 15 repetitions with practice. You can use light weights to increase the work as you grow stronger.

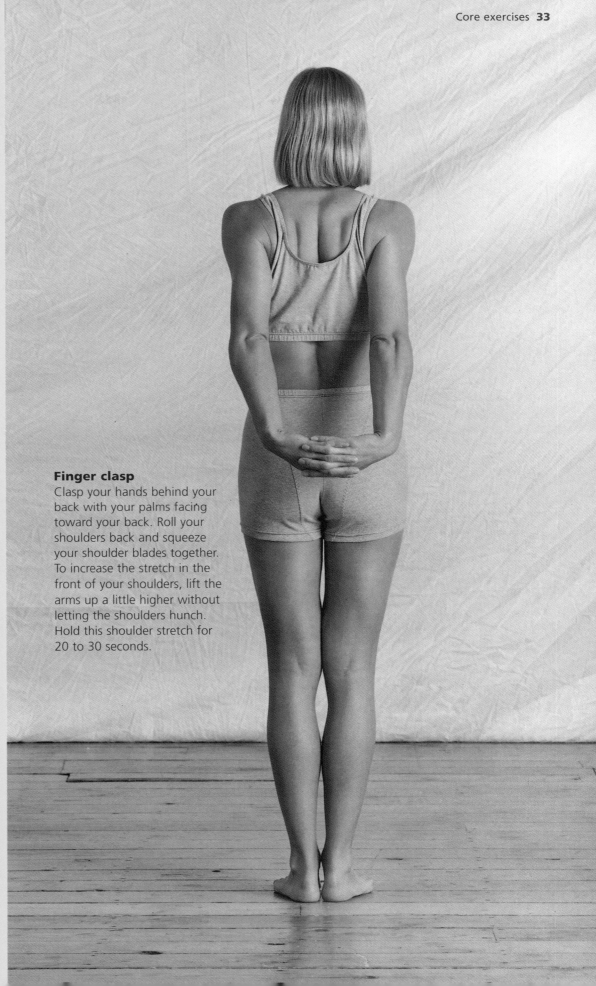

Finger clasp

Clasp your hands behind your back with your palms facing toward your back. Roll your shoulders back and squeeze your shoulder blades together. To increase the stretch in the front of your shoulders, lift the arms up a little higher without letting the shoulders hunch. Hold this shoulder stretch for 20 to 30 seconds.

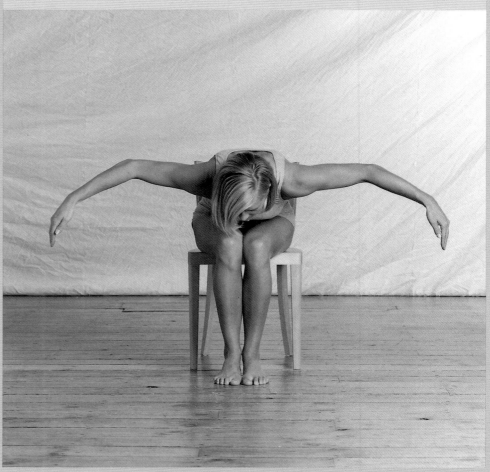

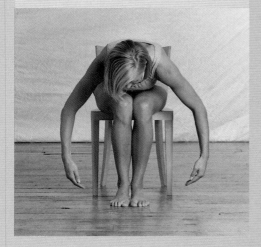

Reverse fly

Working against gravity, you will strengthen your upper back and the backs of your shoulders.

Sitting on a chair, bend over to place your chest on your thighs, keeping your back flat. Begin with your hands by your feet, elbows slightly bent (1). Slowly raise your arms to the side, squeezing your shoulder blades together (2), then lower your arms back to the floor. Repeat 12 times, building up to 20 repetitions. Using light weights will increase the difficulty.

Right angle

Rest your hands shoulders' width apart and at hip height on the back of a chair or against a wall. Bending from the waist, and keeping your legs straight and your back flat, try to create a right angle at your hips. At first, you may have to bend your knees to keep your back flat. Lengthen the backs of your thighs by pushing your buttocks up toward the ceiling, without bending your back. With regular practice, the flexibility in your legs and back will improve. Hold for 20 to 30 seconds.

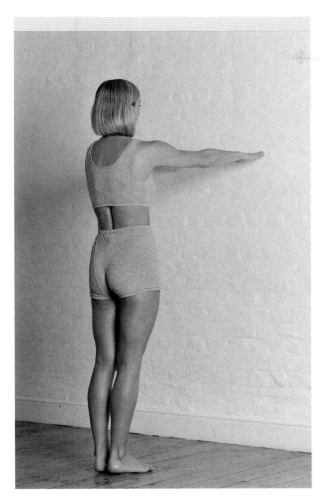

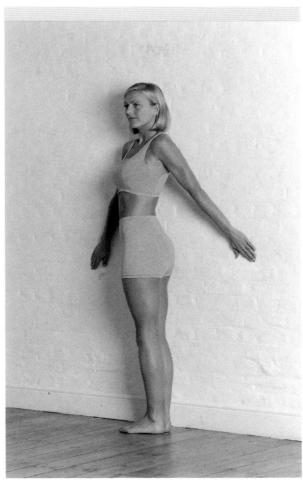

Plank

This simple version of the press-up will strengthen the backs of your upper arms.

Stand at arms' length from a wall with your feet together, tightening your buttocks and drawing your navel to your spine. Place your palms on the wall just below shoulder height and, keeping your elbows close to your rib cage and your back straight, slowly bend your elbows until your nose touches the wall. Straighten your arms, then repeat 15 to 20 times.

Twist from wall

Stand sideways by a wall and, focusing on keeping your hipbones facing forward, slowly twist at the waist, aiming to place your hands on the wall, one either side of you. Make sure your shoulders stay parallel with the floor. Imagine you are separating your navel from your hips. This stretch will mobilize your spine and open your chest. Hold for 20 to 30 seconds, or as long as you are comfortable.

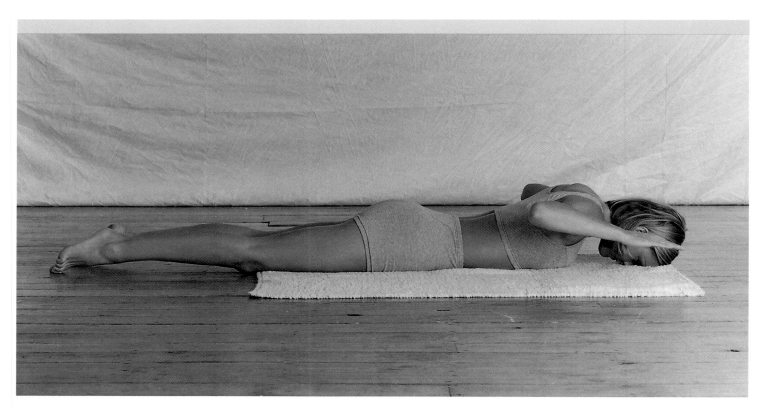

Shoulder blade squeeze

Lying face down on the floor with your feet slightly apart, your elbows bent, and your forearms on the floor, tighten your buttocks and draw your tailbone to the floor and your navel toward your spine. Try to create a gap between your abdominals and the floor, flattening or lengthening the arch in your lower back. Maintaining this alignment, slowly lift your arms and squeeze your shoulder blades together. Hold for a few seconds before relaxing and repeating 10 times.

①

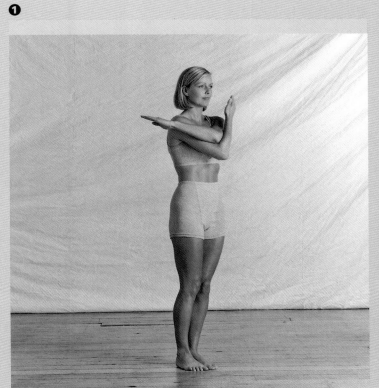

②

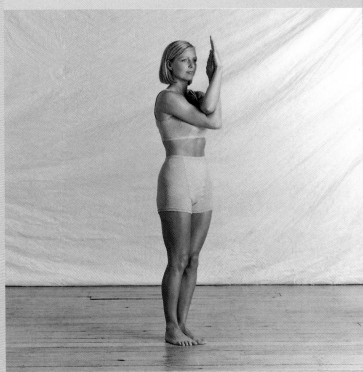

Single arm hug

Take your left arm across your body. Link your right arm under your left and pull your left arm farther across until you feel a stretch over your shoulder blades (1). Try to keep your shoulders away from your ears. To make this stretch more intense, you can wrap your right arm around your left, pressing the fingers of your right hand against your left palm (2).

Waist

Strengthening your abdominals is important not only for your appearance but also for your health. There are no bones in the mid-section of the body, so the abdominal and lower back muscles have sole responsibility for supporting the spine and providing a protective girdle to hold the major internal organs in place. Strength in the muscles of the trunk is vital to maintain good posture and body alignment, and to support the back. With age, the abdominal muscles often weaken and stretch, immobilizing the lower back. A sagging midriff and an exaggerated curve in the lower back look unattractive and place a lot of stress on the lower spine, making it very prone to injury and pain.

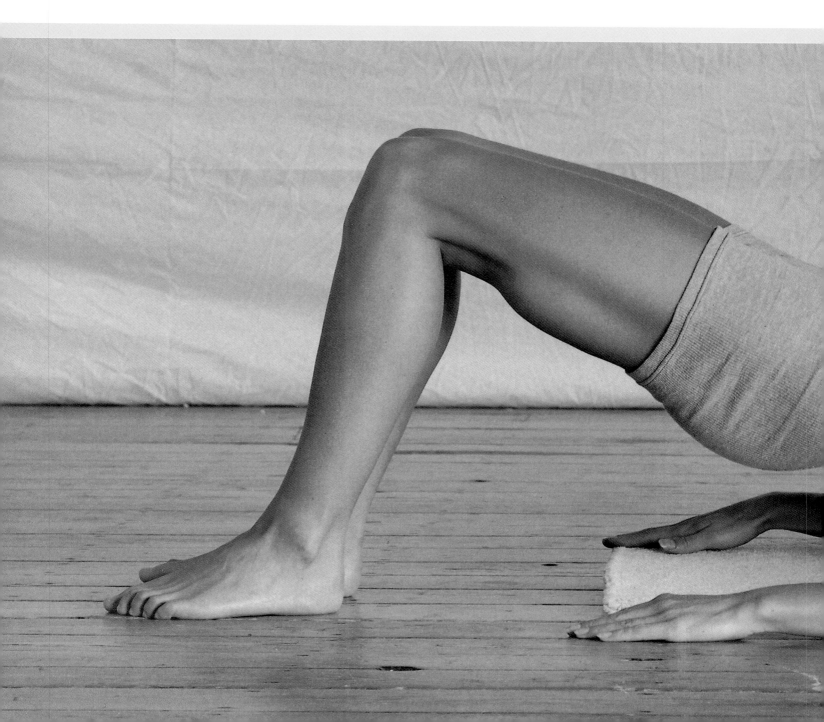

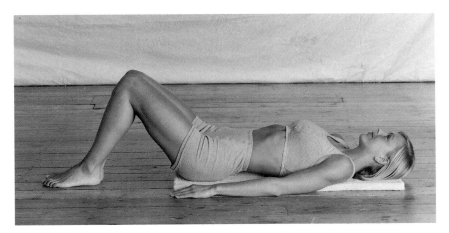

Pelvic tilts

Lie on your back with your knees bent and hips' width apart and your arms by your sides. Try to sink your spine into the floor without straining. Breathing out, scoop in your abdominals, squeeze the backs of your thighs together, and pull up on your pelvic floor muscles as you tilt your pelvis off the floor. As you breathe in, slowly roll back down through the pelvis to the tailbone. Repeat eight to 10 times.

Shoulder bridges

This exercise mobilizes your back. Lying on your back with your knees bent and hips' width apart, and your arms by your sides, squeeze the backs of your thighs together and roll your spine up off the floor one vertebra at a time, starting with the tailbone and moving slowly up. Hold at the top and press your shoulder blades flat into the floor while you open your chest and shoulders. Breathe in, then as you breathe out, slowly uncurl the spine, making each vertebra contact the floor on the way down. Repeat four times, breathing deeply.

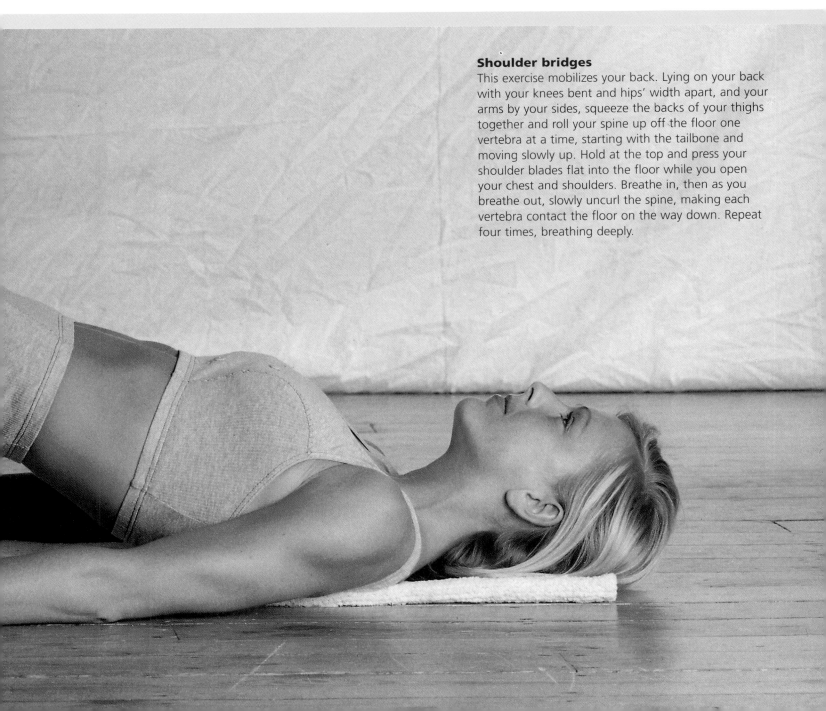

Bicycle

Lie on your back with your knees bent and your hands under your head. Stabilize your back by drawing your navel to your spine and pressing the back of your waist to the floor – as long as you keep your abdominals drawn in, you will not feel any pull in your back. Lift your left leg until the thigh is vertical, then lift your right leg to join it. Slowly lower first one foot, then the other, making sure your lower back remains flat on the floor. Repeat four times.

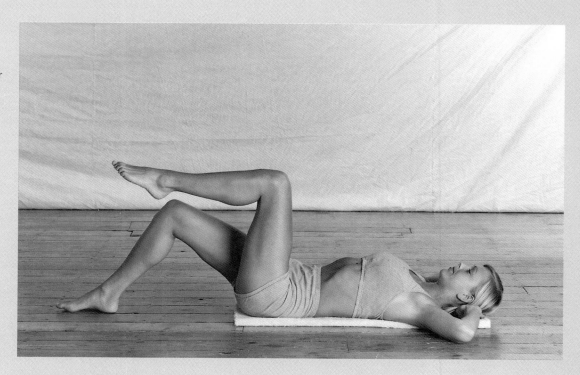

Knee circles

Lie on your back with your knees bent into your chest, clasping your hands lightly around your knees. Moving from the hips, rotate your legs, drawing imaginary circles with your knees that have the small of your back as their center. Make four circles in one direction before reversing and circling the other way.

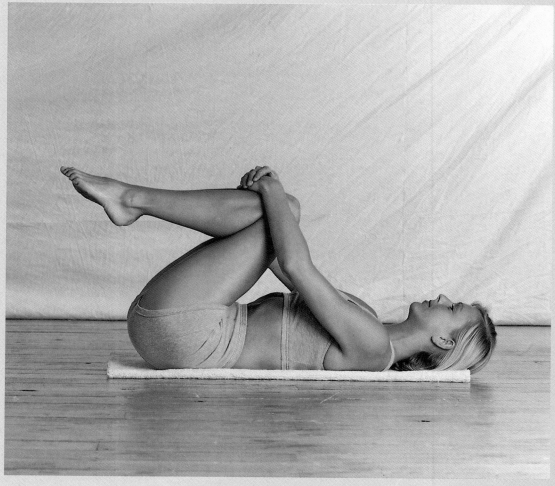

❶

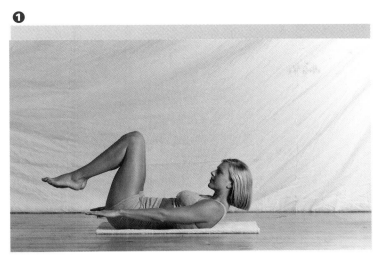

❷

Jackknife

This is an advanced exercise for the abdominals.

  Lying on your back with your knees bent and your arms by your sides, draw your abdominals in firmly and curl your shoulder blades off the floor (1). As you breathe in, unroll through the spine, stretch your arms above your head, and straighten your legs, raising your feet toward the ceiling, making sure your back does not lift from the floor (2). Then, breathing out, bring your arms back to your sides and curl your shoulder blades off the floor. Try to keep your chest open and your neck in line with your spine throughout. Repeat both stages eight times.

Single leg stretch

Lying on your back, bend your right knee, holding it and gently pulling it toward your chest until you feel a stretch in your hip. Press the back of the left thigh to the floor throughout. Hold for 20 to 30 seconds before repeating on the other side.

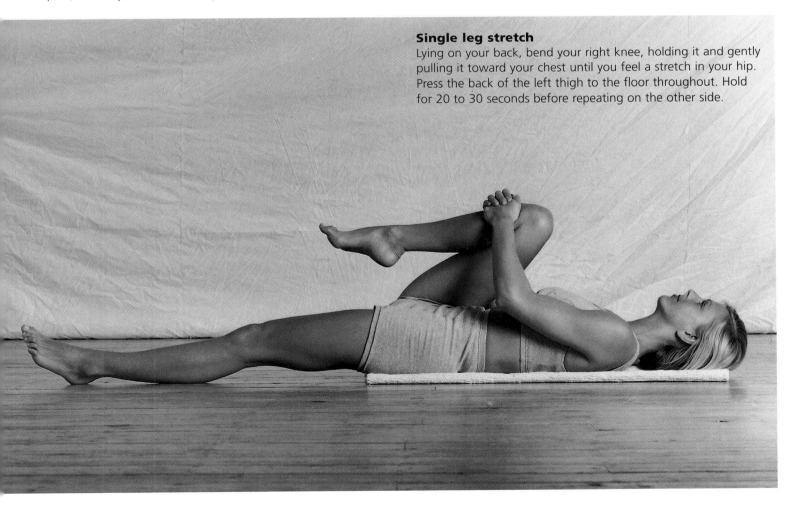

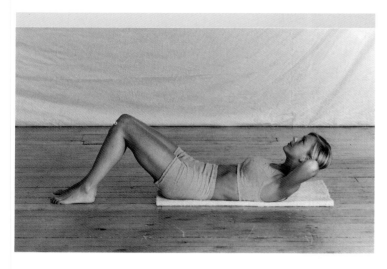

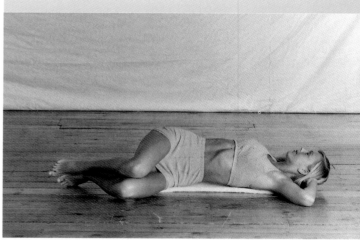

Medicine ball
Lie on your back with your knees bent and your fingers linked behind your head. Anchoring your navel to your spine, breathe out and curl your shoulder blades off the floor. By relaxing your neck muscles and focusing on the contraction of your abdominals, you will be able to avoid the temptation to pull your head up instead of working the key muscles. Relax your head into your hands, and try to curl one more vertebra off the floor. Hold for a count of four, then uncurl. Repeat 10 times.

Double leg hip rolls
Lie on your back with your knees bent, your hands behind your head, and your navel anchored to your spine. As you breathe out, slowly lower your hips and knees to one side, trying to keep your shoulders on the floor. You should feel a stretch in your shoulders. Breathe in as you return to the center. Repeat four times on each side.

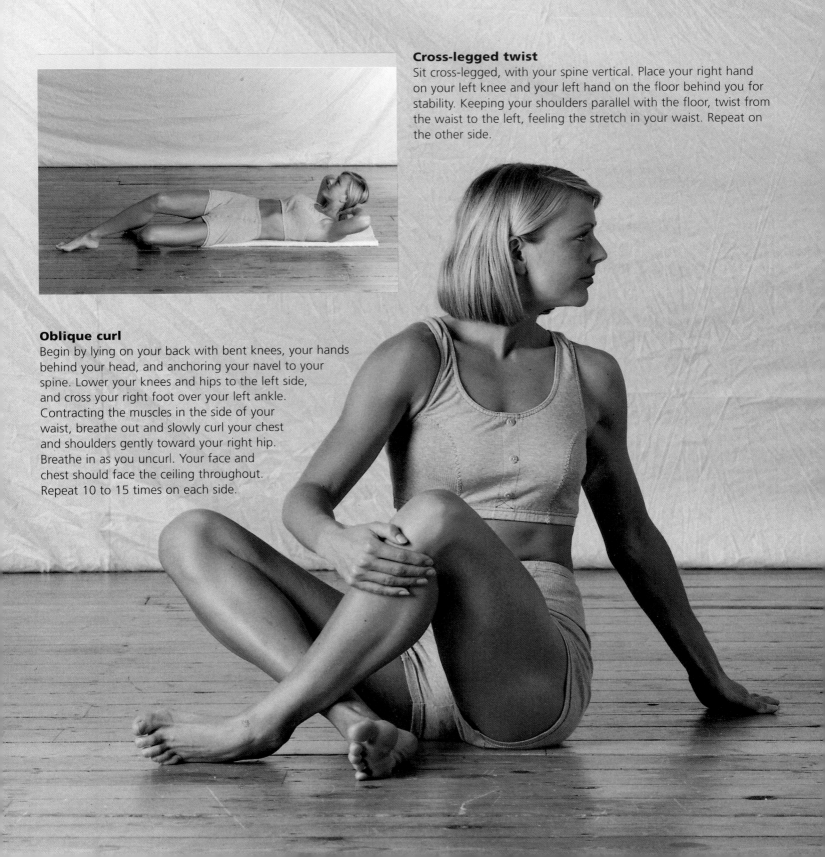

Cross-legged twist

Sit cross-legged, with your spine vertical. Place your right hand on your left knee and your left hand on the floor behind you for stability. Keeping your shoulders parallel with the floor, twist from the waist to the left, feeling the stretch in your waist. Repeat on the other side.

Oblique curl

Begin by lying on your back with bent knees, your hands behind your head, and anchoring your navel to your spine. Lower your knees and hips to the left side, and cross your right foot over your left ankle. Contracting the muscles in the side of your waist, breathe out and slowly curl your chest and shoulders gently toward your right hip. Breathe in as you uncurl. Your face and chest should face the ceiling throughout. Repeat 10 to 15 times on each side.

Diagonal reach

Lying on your back with bent knees, place your left hand behind your head for support and your right hand on the floor by your side. Anchoring your navel to your spine, breathe out and curl the right side of your rib cage toward your left hip, bringing your right arm across your body to your left thigh. Think of lifting your chest, head, and shoulders as one unit up and across your body toward the left thigh, trying to anchor the hips and lower back so you twist diagonally at the waist. Breathe in as you relax back to the floor. Repeat 10 times on each side.

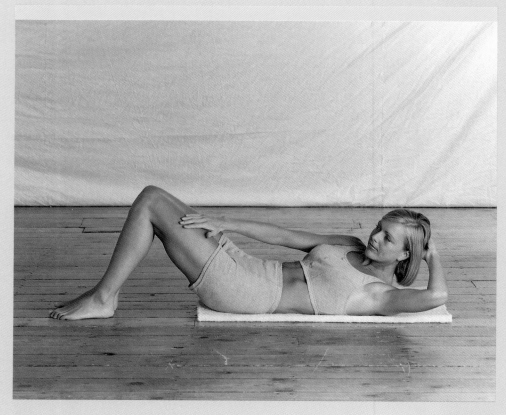

Up-and-over reach

Sit cross-legged with your spine vertical, and place your left hand on the floor, with your shoulder drawn down away from your ear. Bend your spine sideways to the left, reaching over your head with your right arm, keeping both buttocks firmly on the floor, so you feel a stretch in your side. Try not to drop your head forward. Hold for 20 seconds, then relax and repeat on the other side.

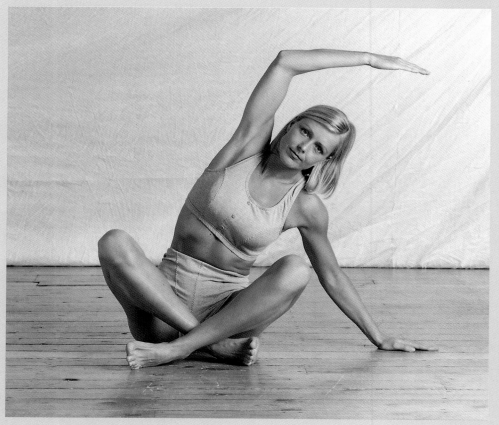

❶

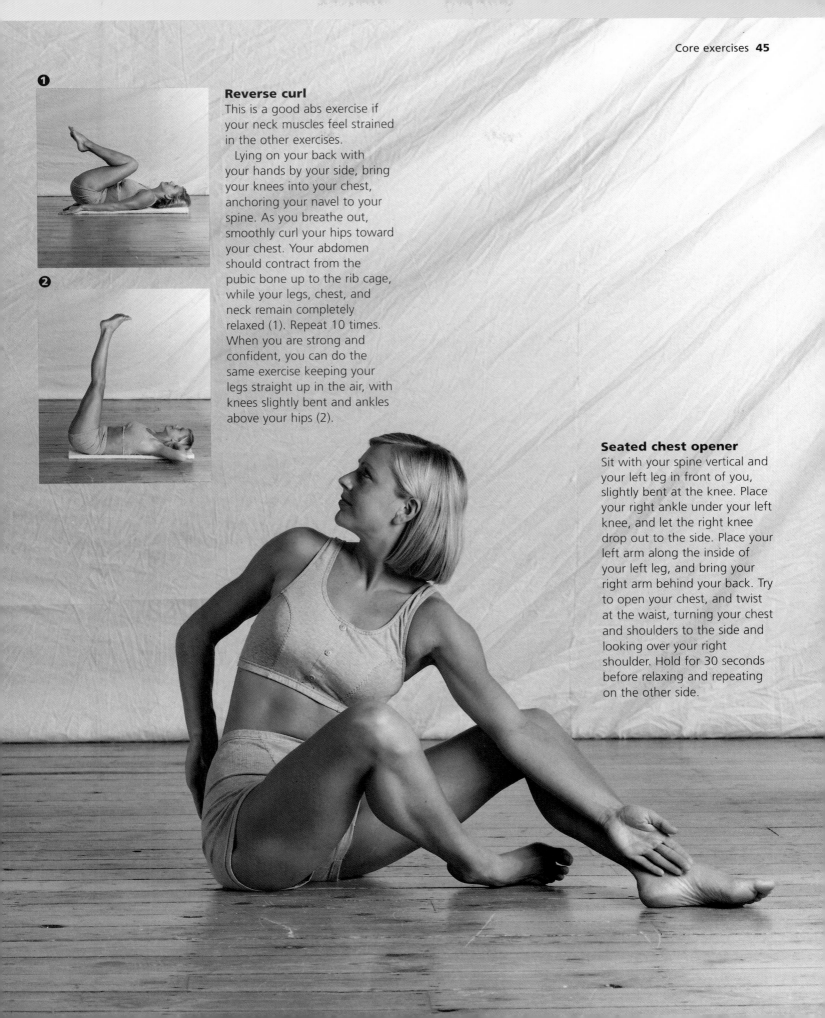

❷

Reverse curl

This is a good abs exercise if your neck muscles feel strained in the other exercises.

Lying on your back with your hands by your side, bring your knees into your chest, anchoring your navel to your spine. As you breathe out, smoothly curl your hips toward your chest. Your abdomen should contract from the pubic bone up to the rib cage, while your legs, chest, and neck remain completely relaxed (1). Repeat 10 times. When you are strong and confident, you can do the same exercise keeping your legs straight up in the air, with knees slightly bent and ankles above your hips (2).

Seated chest opener

Sit with your spine vertical and your left leg in front of you, slightly bent at the knee. Place your right ankle under your left knee, and let the right knee drop out to the side. Place your left arm along the inside of your left leg, and bring your right arm behind your back. Try to open your chest, and twist at the waist, turning your chest and shoulders to the side and looking over your right shoulder. Hold for 30 seconds before relaxing and repeating on the other side.

Warm-ups and cool-downs

Before you start exercising, it is essential to spend five or 10 minutes warming up. Cold muscles are less pliable than warm ones and are more prone to wrenches and strains. Joints can also become stiff and immobile from inactivity. Large, rhythmical movements will raise the temperature of your body and increase the range of motion around your joints. Deep, steady breathing will also help you to clear your mind.

After you have finished exercising, it is just as important to take the time to cool down, gently decreasing the pace and the intensity of your exercise and taking time to relax at the very end.

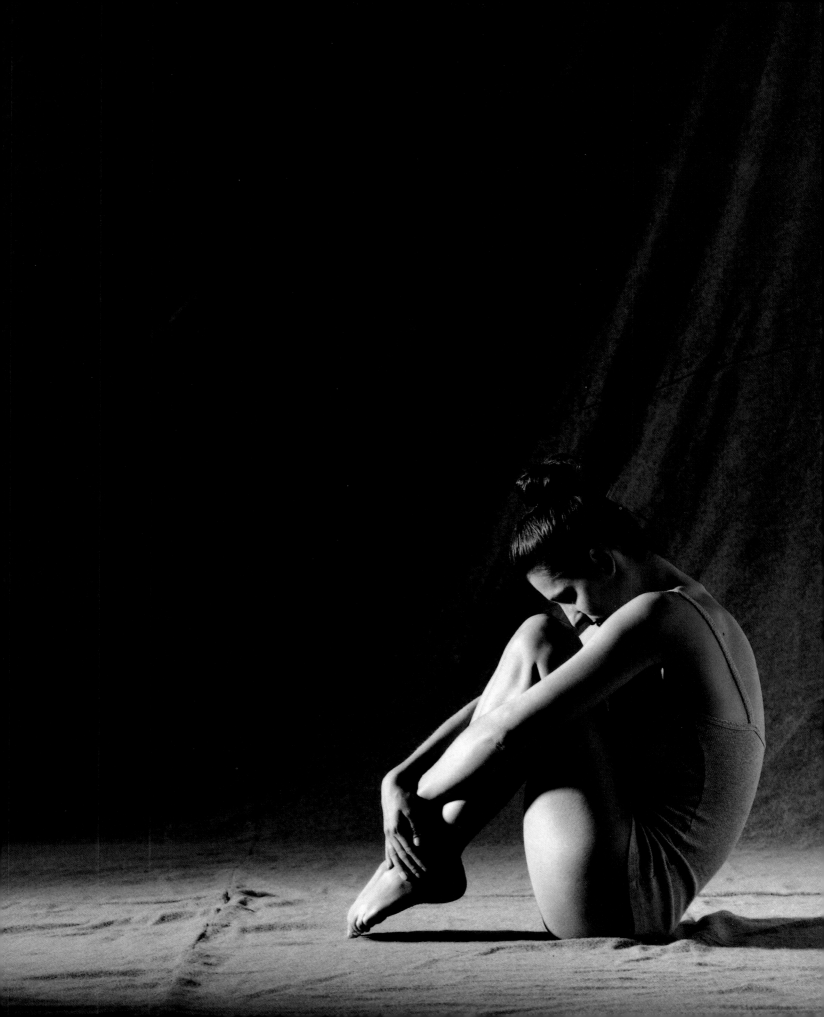

Warm-ups

Before you start any exercise program, it is essential to spend five or ten minutes warming up.

Take your time to perform the warm-up movements slowly and smoothly, focusing on the parts of your body that you are preparing for work. For maximum benefit, it is important to take the joints through a full range of motion without forcing any of the movements. Deep, steady breathing will also help you to clear your mind.

The number of repetitions you perform will depend on how you are feeling at the time of your workout. Do a little extra if you are feeling particularly stiff.

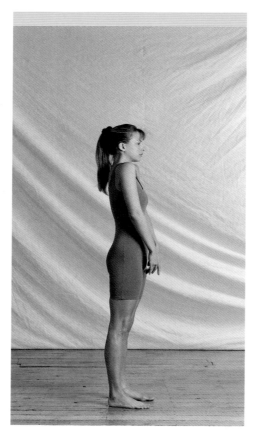

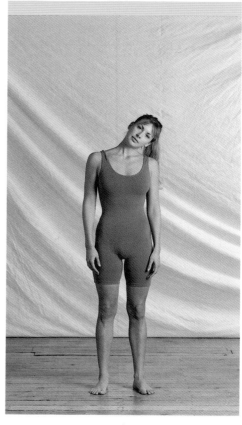

Shoulder circles
Standing comfortably with good posture, bring your shoulders first forward, then up to your ears, and then back so you squeeze your shoulder blades together. Make sure that your neck does not drop forward and that your rib cage does not protrude: you can watch yourself in a mirror if that helps. Repeat eight times before reversing the action.

Neck tilt
Standing upright, tilt your head to one side, stretching the side of your neck, then straighten your head before tilting to the other side. Repeat four times on each side.

❶ **❷**

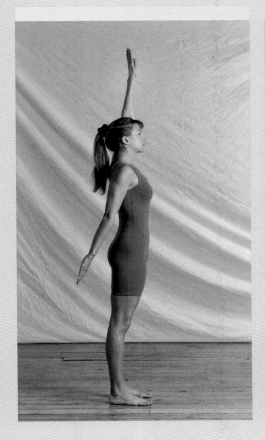

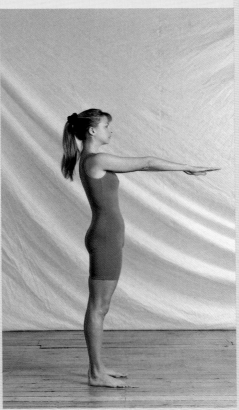

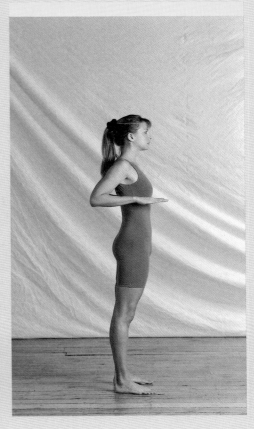

Single arm reach

Keeping your arms straight, reach your left arm up to the ceiling as you extend your right arm behind you. Make sure your body doesn't twist. Repeat eight times before switching arms.

Chest opener

Beginning in an upright position with your arms straight in front of you at chest height (1), squeeze your elbows back behind the rib cage to open up the chest and shoulders (2). Repeat eight times, keeping the movement slow and even.

Full arm circles

Standing with good posture, circle your arms forward, then up and over the head, and finally behind the body. Keep your arms straight but do not lock your elbows, and make the movement as wide and free as possible. Repeat eight times in one direction before reversing the movement.

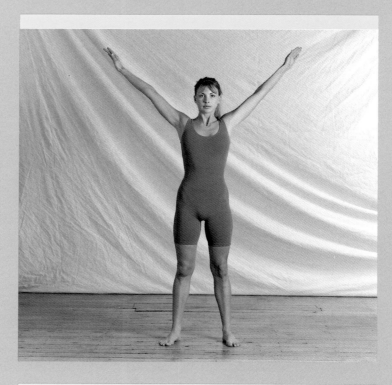

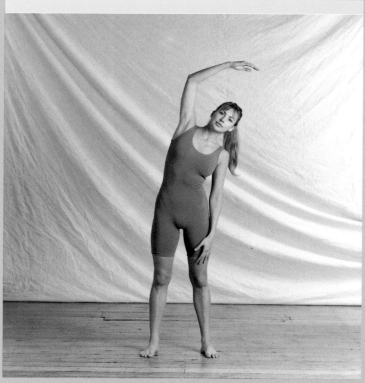

Side reach

Standing with your feet shoulders' width apart, rest your left hand on your thigh and reach up and over your head with your right hand. As you bend to the left, you will stretch the muscles in your right side. Repeat four times on each side.

Torso twists

As you stand with your feet shoulders' width apart and your arms slightly bent at the elbow, twist your upper body smoothly and with control to one side then the other, keeping your hips facing forward. Repeat eight times on each side.

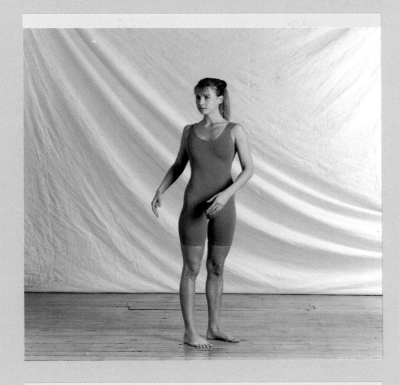

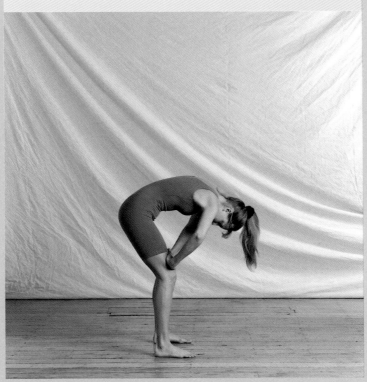

Contractions

Begin standing with your feet hips' width apart, knees bent, and your hands on your thighs. First, round your back, letting your chin drop to your chest, then ripple through your spine until you return to a flat back. This will loosen your back muscles and mobilize your spine. Repeat eight times.

Cool-downs

By gently stretching the muscles you have worked, you will minimize soreness and allow your body temperature to return to normal. Aim to hold each stretch for the recommended time, but be careful not to force or strain your body in any way.

With these cool-down exercises, you will open the chest and shoulder girdle to ensure that your lungs have the space to breathe freely and easily. Your spine should feel free and your abdominals lengthened but firm. Stretching your neck and upper back will help to ease any lingering stiffness and leave your whole body feeling relaxed and free of tension.

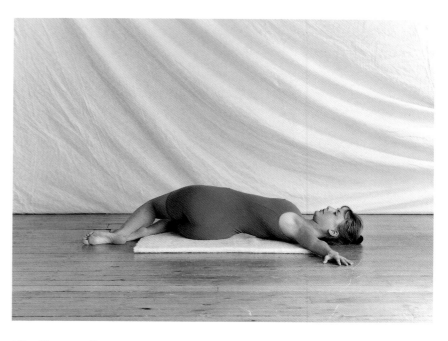

Hip flexor tilt

Lie on your back with your knees bent, your arms out to the side, and your navel anchored to your spine. Lower both knees to the right keeping your left shoulder on the floor. Stretch the front of your hip by lifting the left hip and contracting the buttocks. Hold for 20 seconds, then repeat.

❶

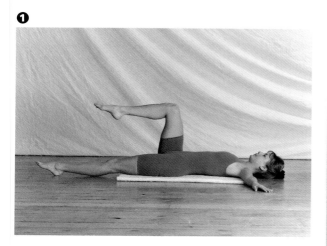

Bent leg cross-over

Lying on your back with your arms straight out to the side at shoulder height, and drawing your shoulder blades down your back, raise your right leg, bending the knee to a right angle, and keeping your left leg straight (1). With your shoulders on the floor, bring your right knee across your body and lower it to the floor (2). Hold the stretch for 30 seconds before repeating on the other side.

❷

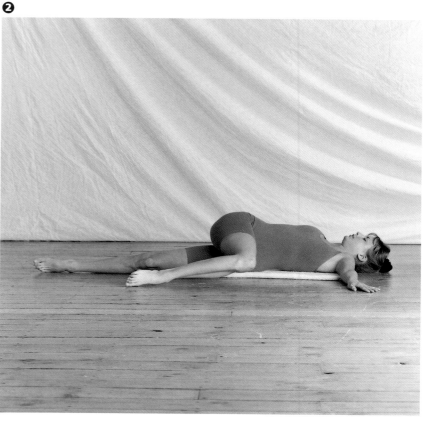

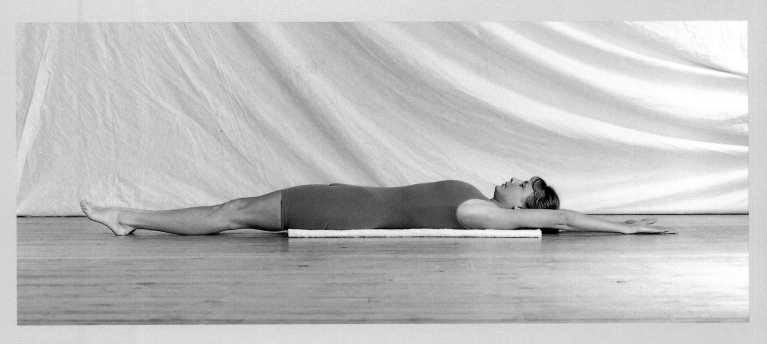

Full-length reach

Lying comfortably on your back, reach up above your head, stretching through your fingertips, at the same time as you stretch your legs down and away. The aim is to move your fingers and your toes as far away from each other as possible. Hold for 30 seconds, breathing deeply throughout, as you rid your body of stress and tension.

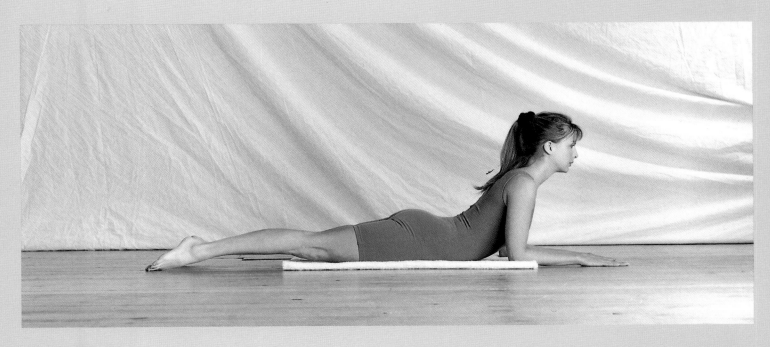

Sphinx stretch

Lying on your stomach, place your arms by your sides with the elbows bent and the forearms parallel to your body. As you contract your buttocks to draw your tailbone to the floor, raise your upper body off the floor. Looking forward, open your chest and shoulders until you feel a stretch through the front of your body. Keep your neck aligned with your spine, and fix your eyes on one point in front of you for concentration. Breathing deeply, hold for 30 seconds.

Cat stretch
Kneeling, with your hands under your shoulders and your knees under your hips, round your back and let your head relax down, then arch your back and lift your head up to look straight ahead, rippling through each vertebra as you do so. Repeat four times.

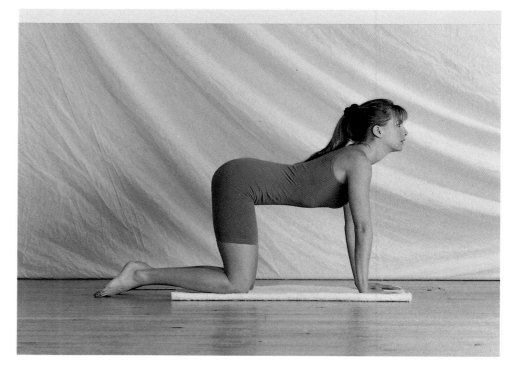

Prayer mat
Sitting back on your heels with your arms stretched forward, shoulders' width apart, slide forward, keeping your arms straight, until your hips are just behind your knees. With your spine long and your navel drawn in toward your spine, drop your forehead and nose to the floor. As you do, you will feel a stretch in your shoulders and armpits.

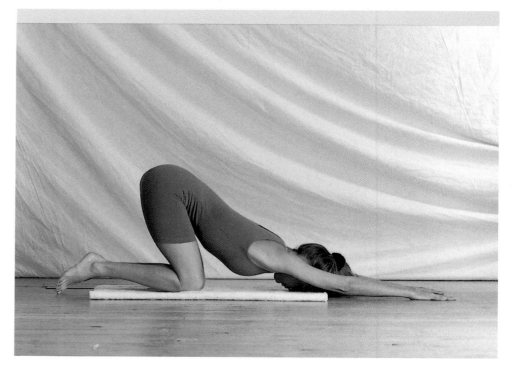

Hand clasp

Sitting back on your heels, clasp your hands behind you with your palms touching, and squeeze your shoulder blades to stretch your chest. To increase the stretch, you can bend forward and raise your arms up and away from your body. If you cannot clasp your hands together, start by clasping your fingers.

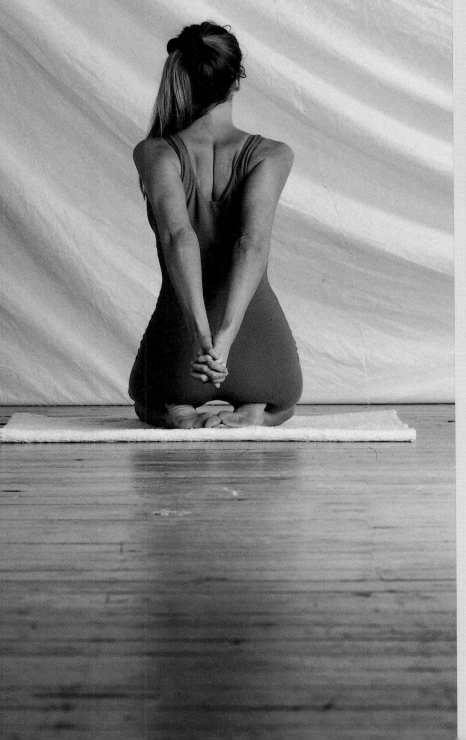

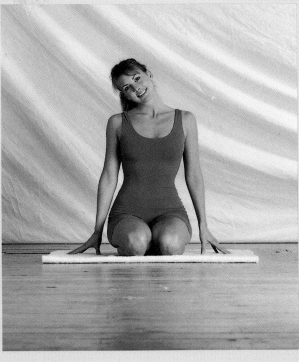

Half neck circles

Sitting on your heels with good posture, drop your head to the right so your ear approaches your shoulder, then move it slowly around to the front until your chin is against your chest, and continue the movement through until your left ear approaches your left shoulder. Return to the center, then repeat in the opposite direction. Don't circle your head backward because this may strain the vertebrae in your neck.

Total body workout

These exercises targeting the hips, thighs, buttocks, and back complement the core chest and shoulder exercises, and they will help to strengthen the whole body. Imbalances in the hips and thighs can tilt the pelvis out of alignment, forcing the spine out of its natural curve. Strong legs also protect the hip and knee joints.

The standing exercises here are compound – they strengthen several muscles in the leg at once. These are backed up by targeted exercises that will strengthen individual muscles.

When you are starting out, select one compound exercise and one isolation exercise each for the inner, outer, front, and back of your thighs. As you become stronger, you will be able to complete the whole set.

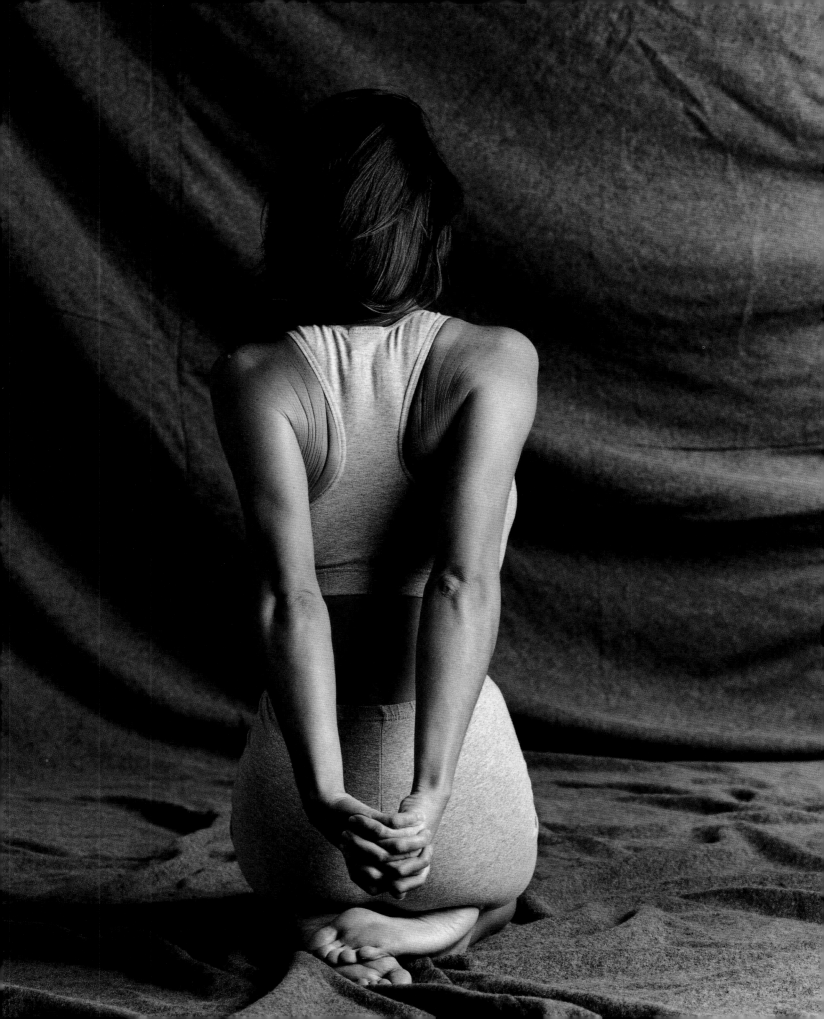

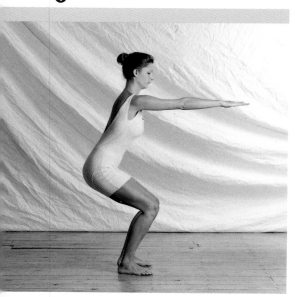

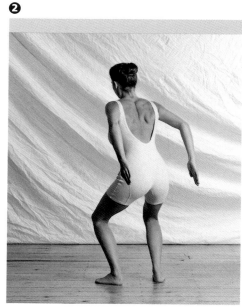

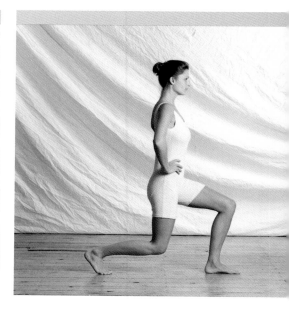

Squat

This is a good all-over exercise for the hip and thigh area. Standing with your feet shoulders' width apart and your feet and knees facing forward, slowly squat, bringing your hips back and down and raising your arms to shoulder height to help your balance. Keep your back flat and your chest open throughout (1). As your legs strengthen, you will be able to lower your body until your thighs are parallel to the floor.

As you return to standing, focus on contracting the buttocks without tucking your pelvis, so you work the hips without putting stress on your knees. Repeat between 10 and 20 times.

For an advanced variation, requiring more coordination and balance, bring your arms behind your body as if you would eventually squeeze the backs of your arms together (2), instead of bringing them up in front of you.

Lunge and tilt

Bending your left knee, place your left foot in front of the right so your shin is vertical to the floor and your thigh is horizontal. As you pull your abdominals in and press your pelvis forward, you will feel a stretch in the front of your right hip and thigh. Hold for 30 seconds before changing legs.

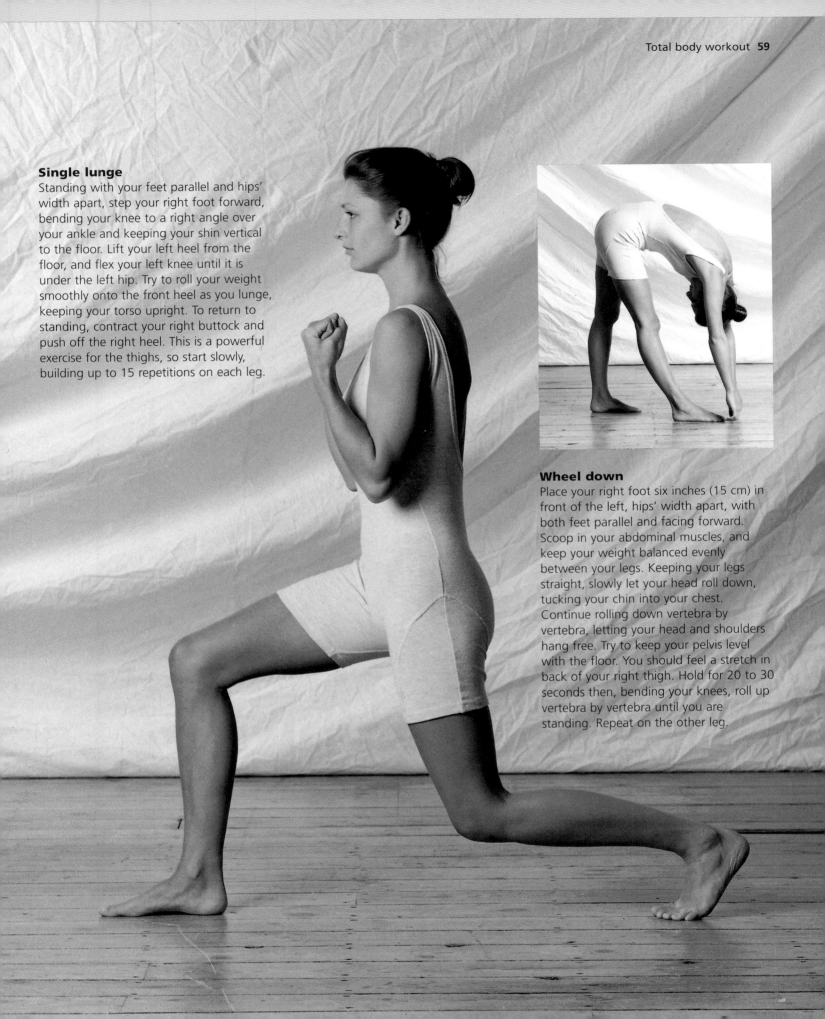

Single lunge

Standing with your feet parallel and hips' width apart, step your right foot forward, bending your knee to a right angle over your ankle and keeping your shin vertical to the floor. Lift your left heel from the floor, and flex your left knee until it is under the left hip. Try to roll your weight smoothly onto the front heel as you lunge, keeping your torso upright. To return to standing, contract your right buttock and push off the right heel. This is a powerful exercise for the thighs, so start slowly, building up to 15 repetitions on each leg.

Wheel down

Place your right foot six inches (15 cm) in front of the left, hips' width apart, with both feet parallel and facing forward. Scoop in your abdominal muscles, and keep your weight balanced evenly between your legs. Keeping your legs straight, slowly let your head roll down, tucking your chin into your chest. Continue rolling down vertebra by vertebra, letting your head and shoulders hang free. Try to keep your pelvis level with the floor. You should feel a stretch in back of your right thigh. Hold for 20 to 30 seconds then, bending your knees, roll up vertebra by vertebra until you are standing. Repeat on the other leg.

Heel raise plié

Stand with your feet wider than shoulders' width apart, feet and knees turned out (1). Raise your right heel, keeping your weight evenly divided over both feet (2). With your spine vertical, bend your knees, keeping them lined up over your feet. Try to squeeze your knees back and out by contracting your buttocks before you carefully straighten up. Repeat on the other side.

This exercise requires good flexibility in the hip joint – if your knees are dropping inward, bring your feet closer together to build up enough flexibility and strength to do the full exercise with good form. Repeat between 10 and 20 times.

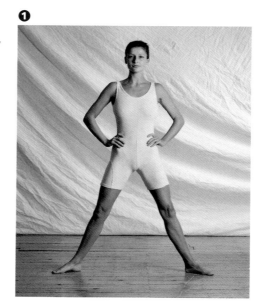
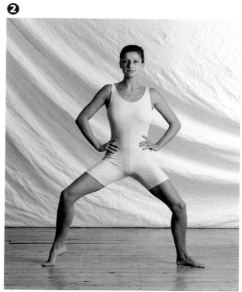

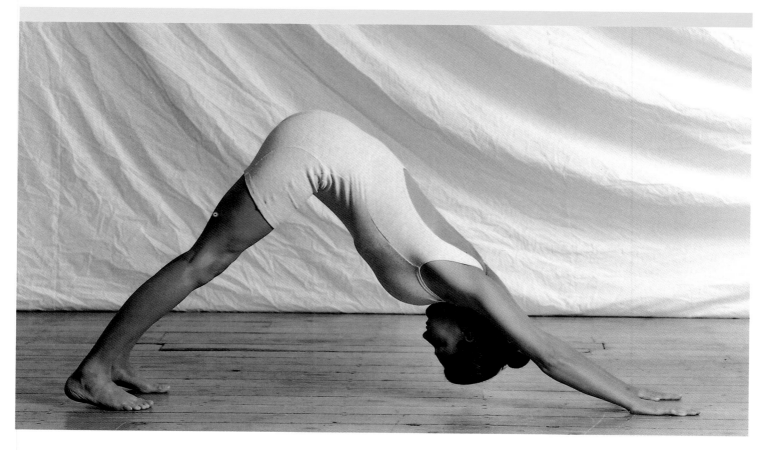

Diamond dog

Roll down through your spine to place your hands on the floor, shoulders' width apart. Walk your hands forward, keeping your legs and arms straight, until you are in a pyramid shape. Press your palms into the floor and try to press your heels to the ground, feeling an increased stretch through the backs of your legs. Letting your head hang free, hold for 20 to 30 seconds, breathing deeply into the stretch and thinking about raising your tailbone higher from the floor, before lowering yourself to your hands and knees and sitting back onto your heels. If you have weak shoulders, you should avoid this stretch.

Freestyle kick

Lying on your stomach with your feet hips' width apart and your forehead resting on your hands, draw your tailbone to the floor by contracting your buttocks, and pull in your abdominals to flatten out your lower back a little. Lift one leg only a little off the floor, keeping your pelvis anchored to the floor and feeling the back of the thighs and the buttocks working: if you lift your leg too high, you will feel it in your lower back. You should relax your upper body completely, focusing on the backs of the thighs. Repeat eight to 20 times on each leg.

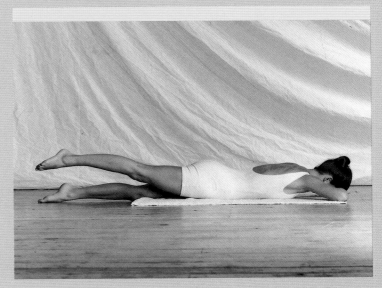

Lying quad stretch

Lying on your stomach with your head turned to the right, your knees together, and your arms relaxed by your sides, hold your left foot or ankle with your left hand, your elbow bent out to the side, and draw the heel toward the right buttock. Pull in your abdominals, and draw your tailbone to the floor by contracting your buttocks. You should feel a strong stretch in the front of your thigh. Hold the stretch for 30 seconds, letting your shoulders and neck relax completely, before changing legs.

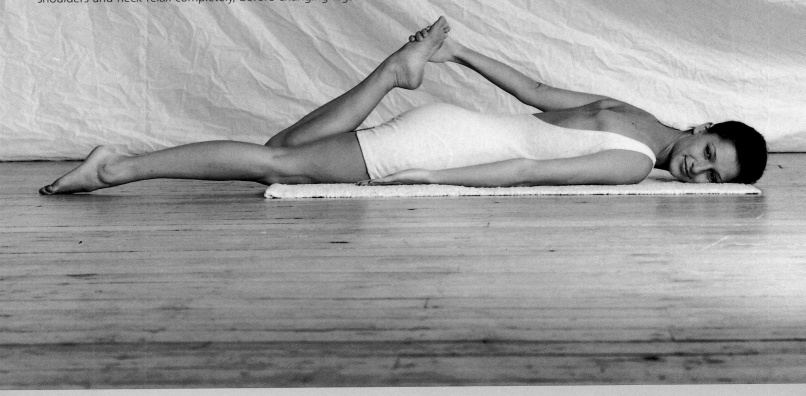

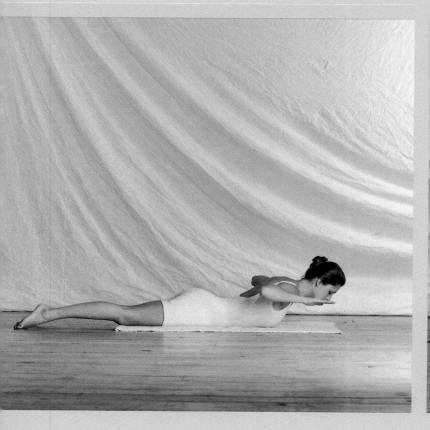

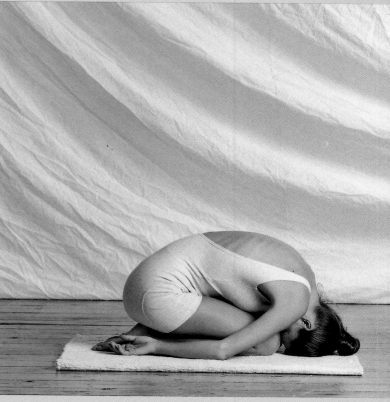

Back extension
Lie face down with your feet hips' width apart and your arms by your sides bent at the elbows, and draw your tailbone to the floor by contracting your buttocks. Keeping the back of your neck long and your eyes facing the floor, breathe in and raise your chest a little off the ground until you feel your lower back muscles contract. Breathe out as you lower yourself back to the floor. Your spine should lengthen and lift, but your feet should stay anchored to the floor throughout. Repeat eight times, building up to 20 repetitions as you become stronger.

Once your back has strengthened, you can place your hands under your forehead to increase the intensity of the exercise.

Sit back
Sit back into your heels, lowering your upper body so your chest rests on your thighs, and place your arms by your sides. Relax completely, releasing any tension in your spine.

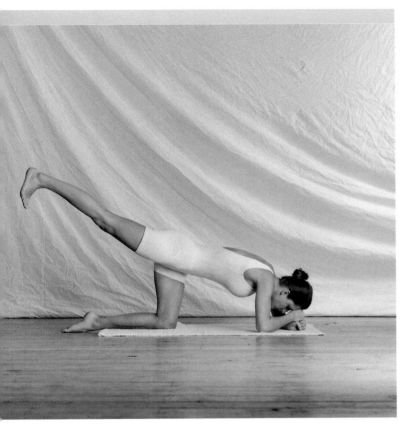

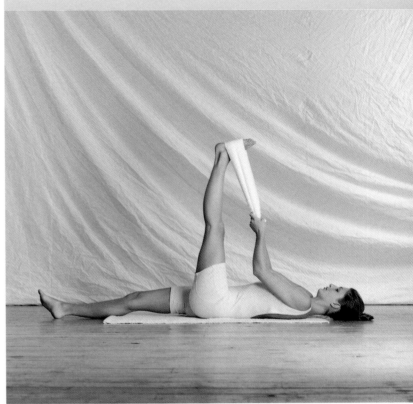

Hamstring curl

On all fours, place your elbows under your shoulders and your knees under your hips. Scoop in your abdominals and keep your back strong and straight. Extend your right leg and lift it straight up and back, without dropping your body to the left side. Slowly curl the heel toward your hip, concentrating on squeezing the back of your thigh. Extend your leg, straightening it, before repeating 15 to 20 times on each leg. When you are confident of the strength and stability of your torso, you can support your forehead on your fists.

Hamstring stretch

Lying comfortably on your back with your legs straight in front of you, draw your left leg toward your chest and place a towel around the ball of your foot. Take a towel end in each hand and straighten your leg without locking your knee joint, pressing the back of your right thigh into the floor to ensure that your hips don't lift. You should feel a strong stretch in the back of your thigh; to stretch your calf, flex your foot toward your shin. You are aiming to get the left leg vertical with the floor without straining. Hold for 30 seconds, then relax before repeating on the other leg.

Abductor raise

Lie on your left side with your left arm stretched out and your right hand placed firmly on the floor in front of you for support. Bend your left leg to 45°, and keep your right leg aligned with your body. Stabilizing your torso by pulling in your abdominals and creating a gap between your waist and the floor, slowly raise your top leg, trying to tighten the muscles in the side of your hip. Squeeze these muscles for a count of two, then lower the leg.

If you find it difficult to isolate the hip muscles, place one hand on your top hipbone and check that there is no movement of the hipbone toward the ribs. The top hipbone should stay directly above the bottom one throughout the exercise. This will ensure that you bend at the hip joint and not at the waist.

Repeat 12 times on each side, building up to 20 repetitions as you grow stronger.

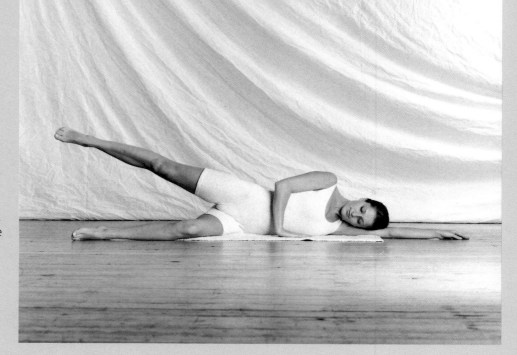

Inner thigh raise

Lie on your left side with your left arm stretched above your head and your right hand placed firmly on the floor in front of you for support. Bend your right leg to a right angle in front of you, and extend your left leg in a straight line with your body. Focusing on the muscles in your inner thigh, lift the left leg off the floor. Hold a few seconds then relax. Repeat between 12 and 20 times on each side.

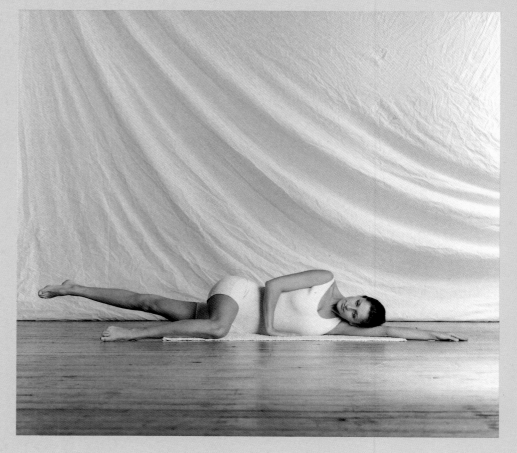

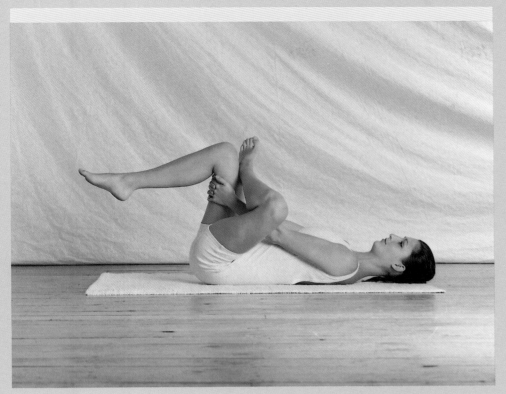

Ankle to knee

Lying on your back with your knees bent and your spine long, place your left ankle on your right knee. With both hands, hold your right thigh, drawing your legs to your chest. Keep your chest and shoulder muscles relaxed and the back of your neck on the floor. You should feel a stretch through the back of your left hip. Hold for 30 seconds, before releasing and changing legs.

When this feels easy, you can extend the right leg vertically to stretch the hamstring at the same time.

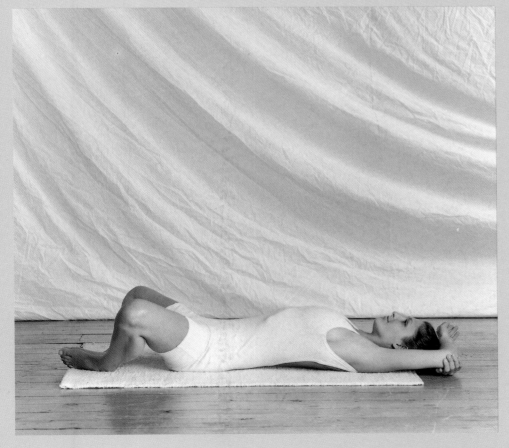

Elbow hold

Lie on your back with your knees bent and the soles of your feet together. Raising your arms above your head, clasp your elbows, trying to press the arms into the floor to stretch the shoulders. At the same time, squeeze your knees toward the floor to stretch your inner thighs. Don't worry if your lower back arches off the floor a little in this stretch. Hold for around 20 to 30 seconds, then relax.

Roll like a ball

Sit with a rounded back, your knees into your chest and your chin tucked in, clasping your hands around your shins as you pull your abdominals in and draw your shoulder blades down your back (1). On a strong out-breath, roll back smoothly through the spine (2) onto your shoulders (3), then, with the same momentum, roll straight back up to sitting.

   Do not throw your head back to initiate the roll – your whole body should be involved in the movement. As your back loosens up, you should feel each vertebra making contact with the mat. Repeat four times.

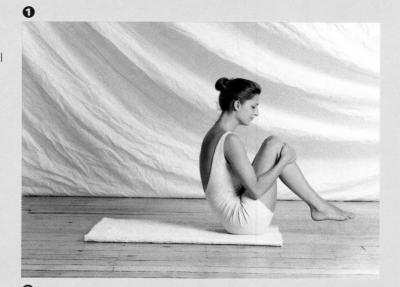

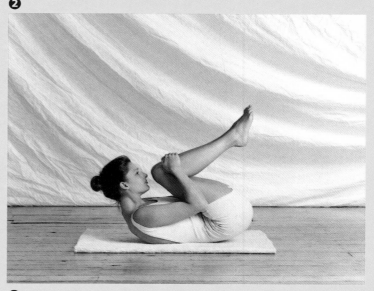

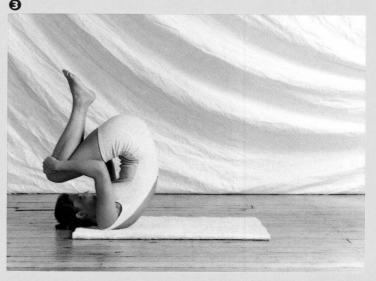

①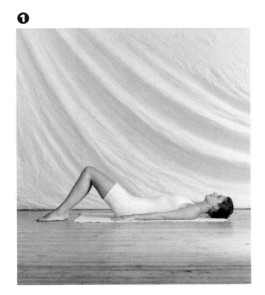

②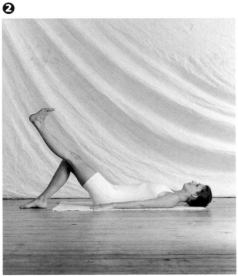

Toe flex and quad extension

Lie on your back with your knees bent and your arms by your side (1), trying to keep the length of your spine, from your tailbone to the top of your head, in contact with the floor. Extend your left leg to 45°, and alternatively flex (2) and point your foot, before lowering your leg to the starting position. Repeat 12 to 20 times on each leg.

Wheel up

With your feet hips' width apart and your knees slightly bent, let your head and shoulders hang free. Scoop in your abdominals, and slowly roll up through the spine, vertebra by vertebra, leaving your head and shoulders to come back to upright last. This will mobilize your spine and loosen your back muscles.

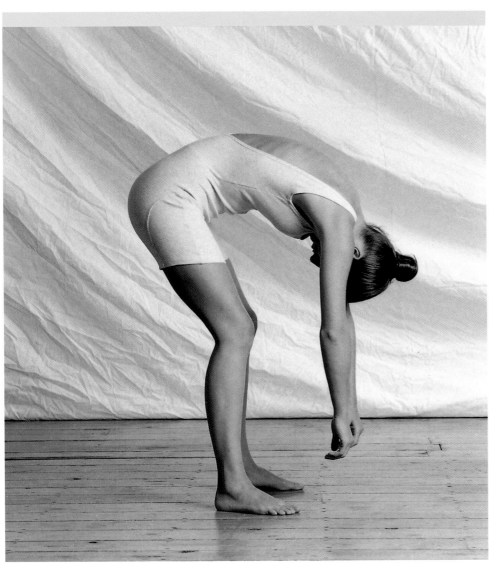

Routines

How you combine exercises to devise a routine will depend on how much time you have, how your day is structured, and what your energy level is at the time. The two sample routines here, which focus on your chest and shoulders, show how you can tailor your choices to suit different situations.

Anything goes as long as you pay attention to working a balance of muscle groups. It is tempting to focus on certain areas of your body – either those you are not happy with, or those you find most satisfying to work – but all your muscles need to be strong and flexible for your body to work efficiently.

Choose exercises that flow smoothly from one to the other, so you do not have to switch positions too often. And assess how you are feeling – let your body be your guide in designing your own routines.

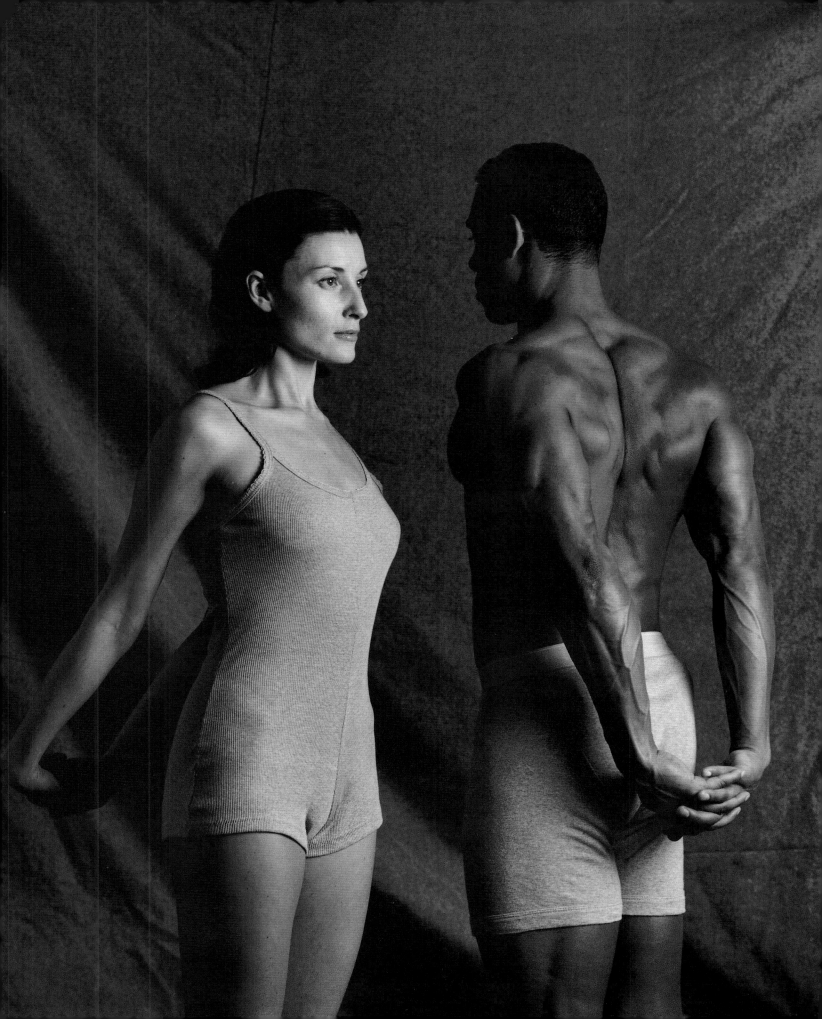

Five-minute loosener

The Five-Minute Loosener is a great way to mobilize your body first thing in the morning or after a long period of inactivity. The gentle stretches energize your muscles and your joints, leaving you feeling refreshed and relaxed. Take your time, breathing deeply and fully through each stretch.

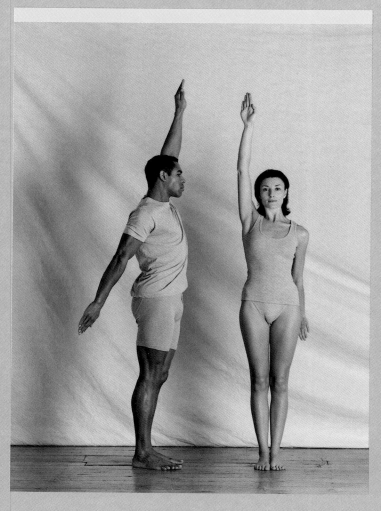

Single arm reach
Without twisting your body, stretch one arm up to the ceiling as you reach the other arm behind you, keeping both arms straight. Repeat eight times on each arm.

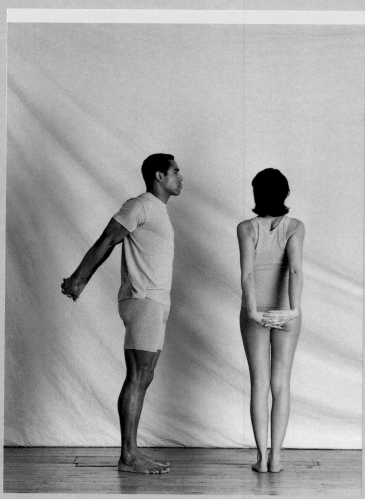

Finger clasp
Interweave your fingers behind your back with your palms facing up. Squeeze your shoulder blades together and stretch your hands back behind you as you raise your arms. Hold for 20 to 30 seconds.

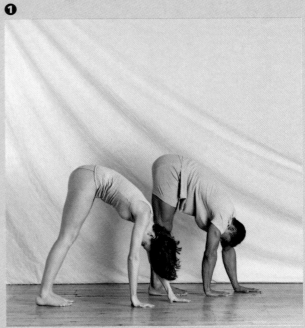

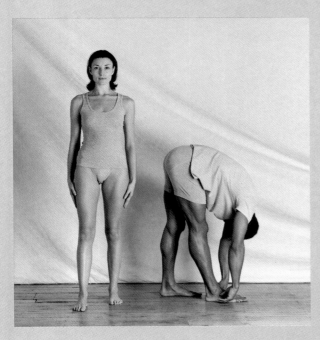

Wheel down

Stand with one leg slightly in front of the other, keeping your feet parallel and your knees slightly bent, and anchor your navel to your spine. Roll down one vertebra at a time starting from the top of the head, letting your head and shoulders hang free, and keeping your hips facing forward. Relax into the stretch, breathing calmly. Pull in your abdominals and bend your knees, then roll smoothly up through the spine, leaving your head and shoulders hanging freely until you return to an upright position. Roll down one more time, and remain there to do the diamond dog.

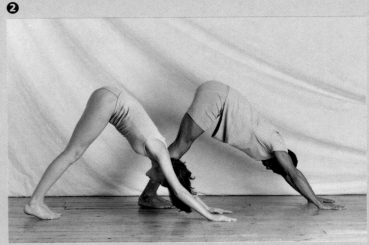

Diamond dog

Flowing from the previous position, walk your hands forward (1), keeping your legs and arms straight, until you are in a pyramid shape. Press your palms into the floor and try to lower your heels to the ground, feeling a stretch through the backs of your legs (2). Letting your head hang free, hold this stretch for 20 to 30 seconds before lowering yourself gently to your hands and knees, then sitting back onto your heels. This stretch may not be suitable if you have weak shoulders.

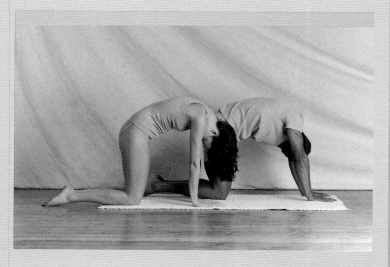

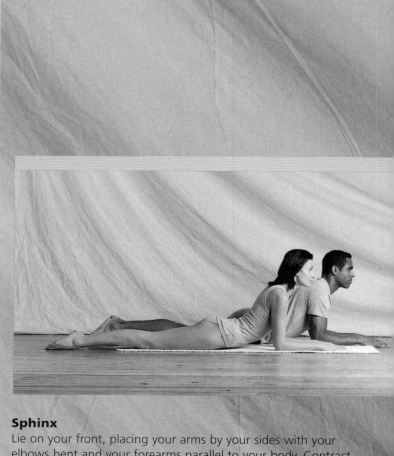

Cat stretch

Resting on your hands and knees, with your hands under your shoulders and your knees under your hips, round your back and let your head relax, then arch your back and lift your head up to look straight ahead, trying to ripple through each vertebra one at a time. Repeat both movements four times.

Sphinx

Lie on your front, placing your arms by your sides with your elbows bent and your forearms parallel to your body. Contract your buttocks to draw your tailbone down, and raise your upper body off the floor. Look straight ahead, lifting your chest and opening your shoulders until you feel a stretch through the front of your body.

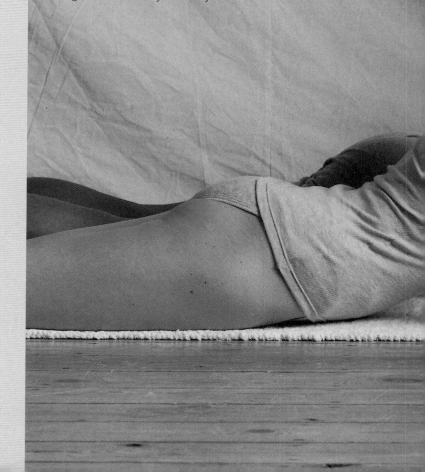

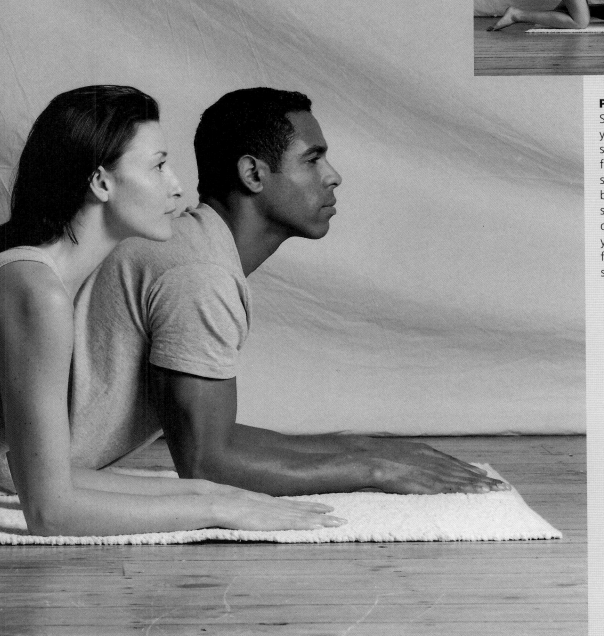

Prayer mat

Sit back on your heels with your arms stretched forward, shoulders' width apart. Slide forward, keeping your arms straight, until your hips are just behind your knees. With your spine long and your navel drawn in to your spine, drop your forehead and nose to the floor to feel a stretch in your shoulders and armpits.

Quick toner

The Quick Toner can be done after playing sports, walking, or running to strengthen some of the muscles not reached by the activity. The movements are more vigorous than the Five-Minute Loosener, so it is important to have warmed up thoroughly before you begin.

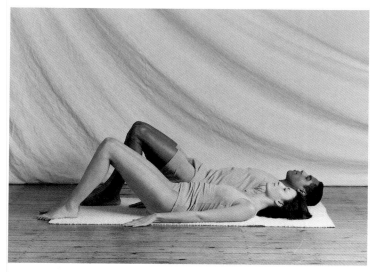

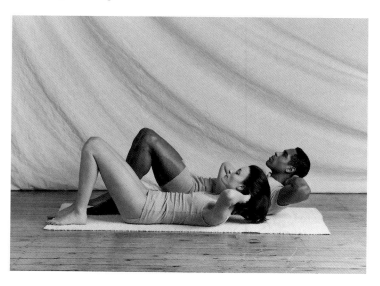

Pelvic tilts

Lie on your back with your knees bent and hips' width apart and your arms by your sides. Try to sink your spine into the floor without straining. Breathing out, draw your navel to your spine and tilt your pelvis off the floor. At the same time, squeeze the backs of the thighs and pull up on the pelvic floor muscles. As you breathe in, slowly roll back down.

With practice, the abdominals, hamstrings, and pelvic floor muscles should do all the work as your buttock and thigh muscles relax. Repeat 10 times, focusing on your breathing.

Medicine ball

Lie on your back with your knees bent and your fingers clasped behind your head. Anchoring your navel to your spine, breathe out and curl your shoulder blades off the floor. By relaxing your neck muscles and focusing on the contraction of your abdominals, you will be able to avoid the temptation to pull your head up instead of working the key muscles. Relax your head into your hands, and try to curl one more vertebra off the floor. Hold for a count of four, then uncurl. Repeat 10 times.

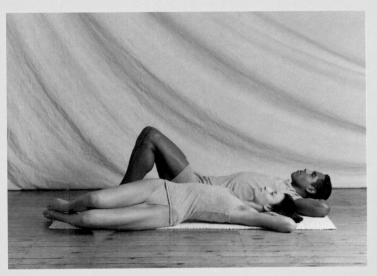

Double leg hip rolls

Lie on your back with your knees bent, your hands behind your head, and your navel anchored to your spine. As you breathe out, slowly lower your hips and knees to one side, trying to keep both shoulders on the floor. You should feel a stretch in your shoulders. Breathe in as you return to the center. Repeat four times on each side.

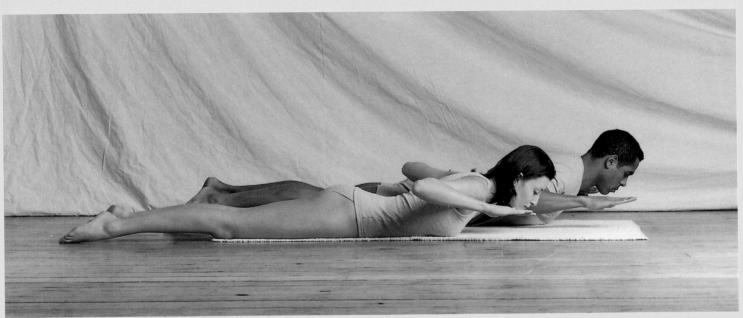

Back extension

Lie face down with your feet hips' width apart and your arms by your side. Draw your tailbone to the floor by contracting your buttocks. Keeping the back of your neck long and your eyes facing the floor, breathe in and raise your chest slightly off the floor until you feel your lower back muscles contract. Breathe out as you lower your chest to the floor. Your spine should lengthen and lift, and your feet should stay anchored to the floor. Once your back has strengthened, you can place your hands under your forehead to increase the intensity. Do between eight to 20 repetitions.

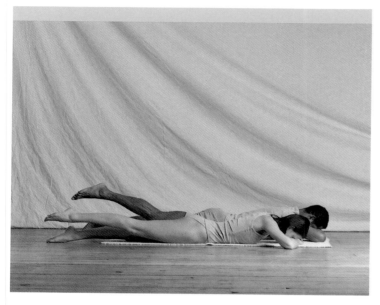

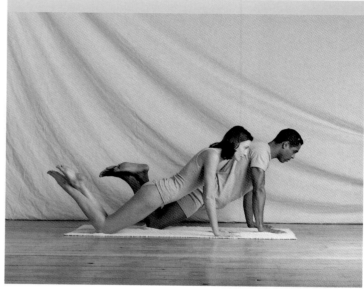

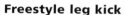

Freestyle leg kick

Lie face down with your feet hips' width apart and your forehead resting on your hands. Draw your tailbone to the floor by contracting your buttocks, and pull in your abdominals to flatten out your lower back slightly. Lift one leg a little off the floor, feeling the back of the thighs and the buttocks working. If you feel it in your lower back, you are lifting your leg too high. Try to relax your upper body completely, focusing on the backs of the thighs doing the work. Repeat eight to 20 times on each leg.

Classic press-up

Starting on your hands and knees, with your hands wider than shoulders' width apart and the fingertips facing forward, establish a straight line from the top of your head through your hips to your knees, and cross your ankles. Keeping your buttocks tight and your navel to your spine, slowly lower your chest toward the floor. Aim to lower your chest all the way to the floor without your body sagging. Raise your body until your elbows are straight again, then repeat up to 20 times.

Bent-over hand clasp

In a kneeling position, clasp your hands behind your back, and press the palms together. Try to turn the backs of your elbows away from you as you squeeze your shoulder blades together. If this feels comfortable, slowly lower your chest to your thighs and try to lift your arms straight up without straining. Hold for 30 seconds, then release. If you find it difficult to clasp your hands, you can begin by clasping your fingers.

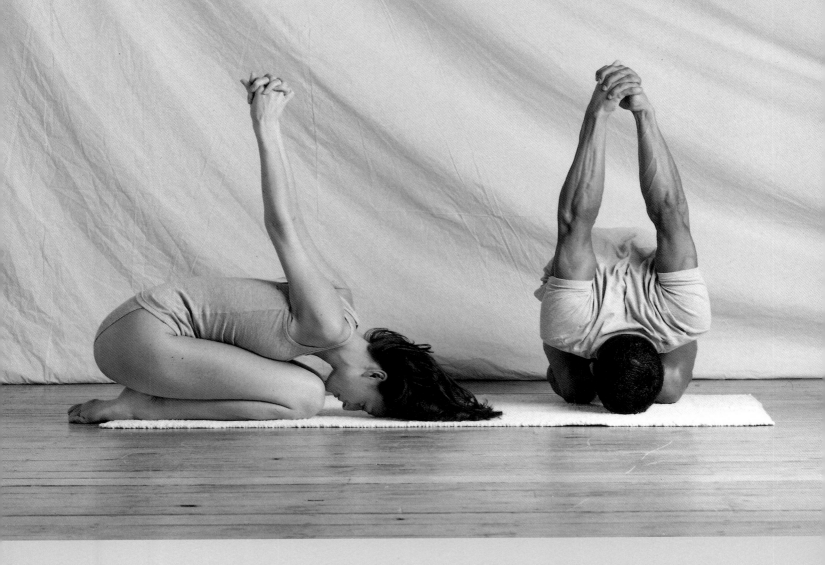

Index

Acknowledgments

Illustrations: Marks Creative

Additional text: Sara Black

Proofreader: Phyllida Hancock

Indexer: Clare Richards

Chair: Montego, by Habitat

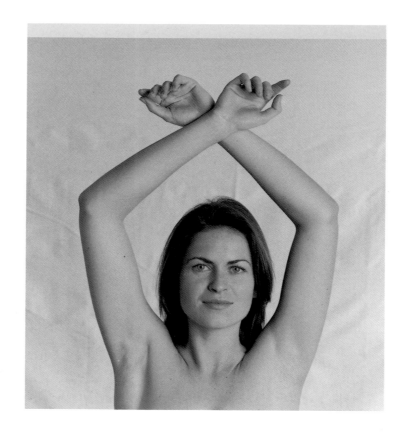